$1.00
(C11) 18/11

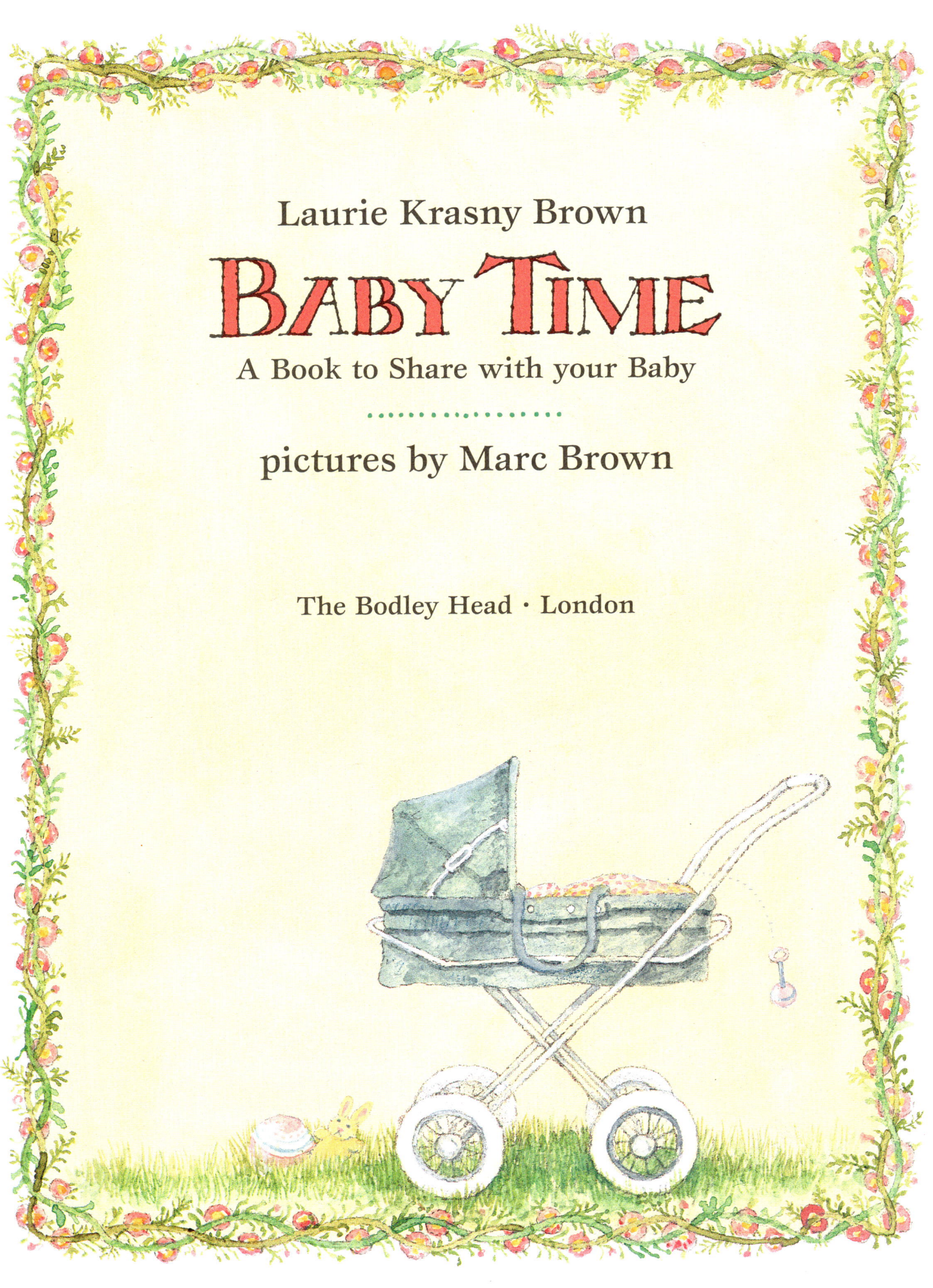

Laurie Krasny Brown

BABY TIME

A Book to Share with your Baby

pictures by Marc Brown

The Bodley Head · London

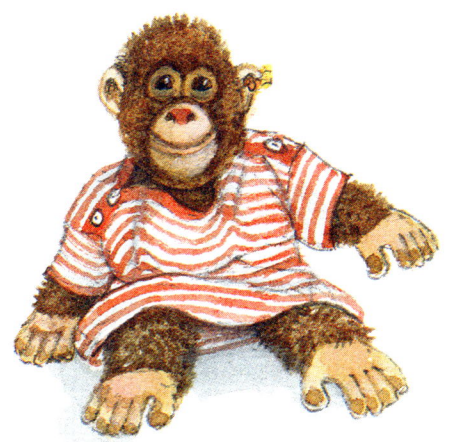

To Eliza, Our Inspiration

British Library Cataloguing in Publication Data
Brown, Laurene Krasny
Baby time 1. Babies. Home care.
I. Title II. Brown, Marc 649'. 122
ISBN 0-370-31294-5

Copyright © 1989 by Laurene Krasny Brown and Marc Brown
All rights reserved under International and Pan-American Copyright Conventions
Printed in the United States by W. A. Krueger for The Bodley Head Children's Books
20 Vauxhall Bridge Road, London SW1V 2SA
First published by Alfred A Knopf, Inc., New York 1989
First published in Great Britain 1990

Special thanks for their generous advice to Dr. Larry Cohan,
pediatrician and teacher of pediatrics,
and Dr. Howard Gardner, professor of education
and adjunct professor of neurology.
The Bodley Head would also like to thank Nancy Stewart
for her kind help.

INTRODUCTION

BABY TIME was inspired by the birth of our daughter. Years of academic training and professional experience in child development did surprisingly little to prepare me for the intense feelings that came with her birth. It seems a privilege—if also the greatest responsibility—to witness daily the gradual unfolding of a new life and have the chance to contribute to that baby's development.

But it's a very personal matter, making the most of the time you and your baby have together. From one day to the next you learn to recognize the kinds of attention your baby needs, and you discover ways to encourage his health, growth, and good spirits. The more confident you become as a parent, the better care you can provide. *Baby Time* is a resource to help you build that confidence.

It helps to have good information about how babies develop. The insights offered here can better enable you to understand how a given form of behaviour reflects your baby's progress. Patience comes much more easily when you can celebrate each tiny achievement as a step along the way to greater maturity.

The best way to develop your intuitive sense is by spending time with your baby, paying good attention to what he does, and taking cues from him. *Baby Time* suggests all kinds of things to do with a baby. Each of the five senses is discussed separately to illustrate how closely your baby's experience is tied to the way things look, sound, smell, taste, feel, and move. Of course, in reality all the senses work together; in fact, one of a baby's developmental tasks is to coordinate the use of the senses.

The activities pictured here were carefully selected to show you how the simplest things you do with your baby can have value and contribute to his growing awareness. Just as important, they present opportunities for having fun together. There is value in that alone.

Best of all, this is a book to enjoy reading *with* your baby. Most babies are ready to look at pictures as soon as they can hold up their heads well, and they especially like seeing pictures of other babies.

So get comfortable with your baby. Some dialogue is suggested, but other comments will no doubt come to mind as you look through the book—you will know best what to say. Skip around and return to pages you both like. When you have finished reading, pick and choose from these ideas and add your own.

Most of all, relax and enjoy your time with your baby!

Laurie Krasny Brown

SIGHT

No sight interests a new baby more than a human face. Let your baby study your face often. Make eye contact with him, and soon he will reward you with his first smile.

It takes babies longer, however, to learn that people continue to exist even when we can't see them. Playing a game of Peekaboo with a baby of six months or older will help your baby learn to understand this.

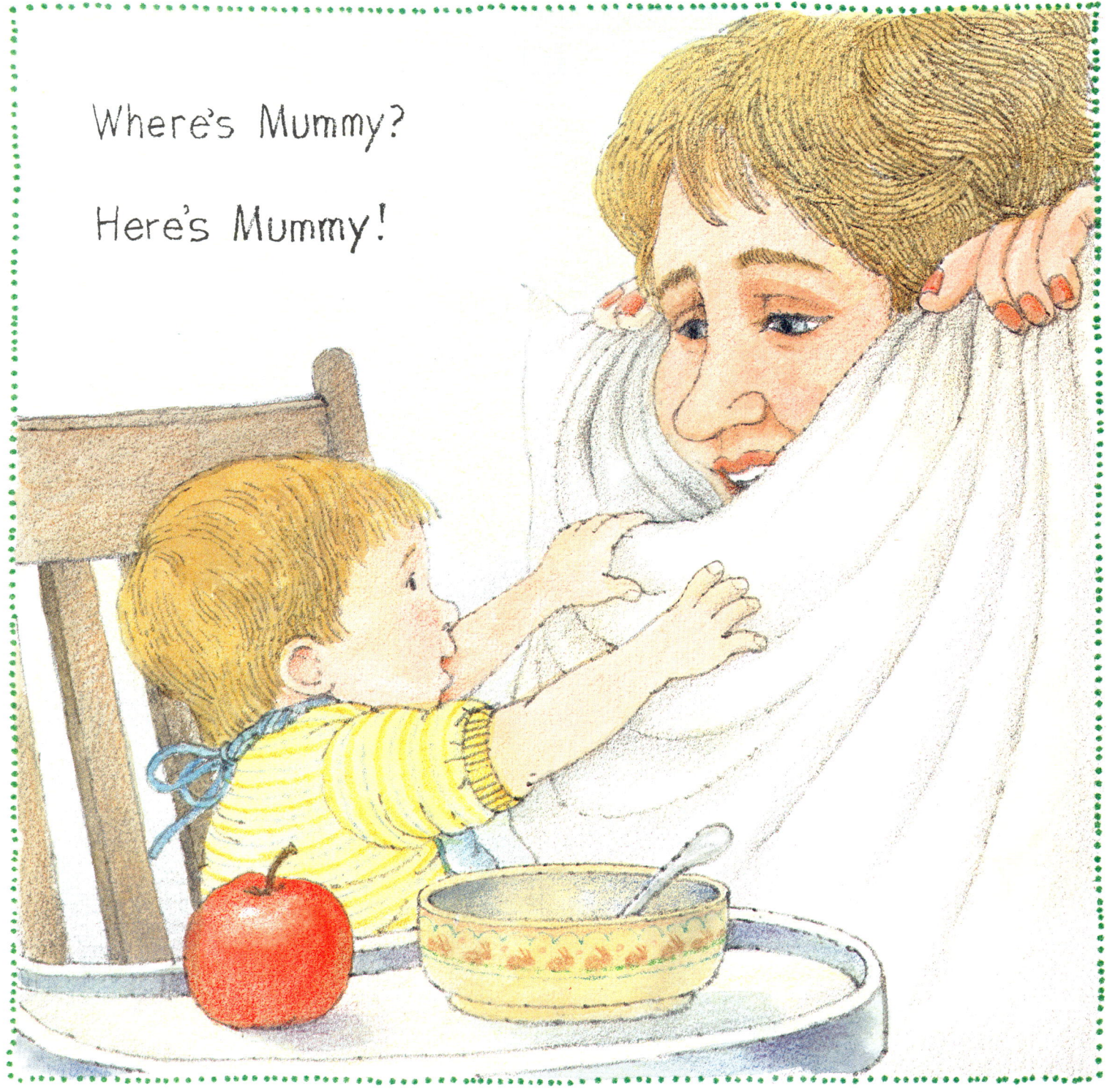

Where's Mummy?

Here's Mummy!

FACES

If you change your appearance, a younger baby, who is still learning to recognize your face, may become confused. Reassure him by trying on and taking off glasses, hats, and the like for him.

Bear in mind that very young babies are nearsighted and can only focus on objects about eight to twelve inches away. This is also—and not incidentally—the distance between a baby's eyes and the face of whoever feeds him.

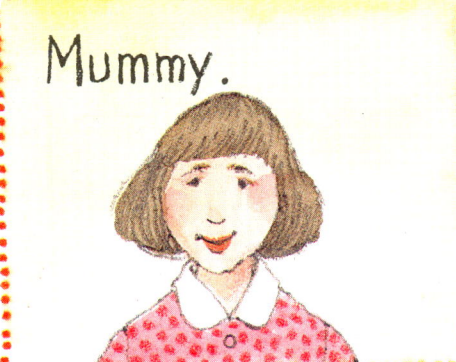
Mummy.

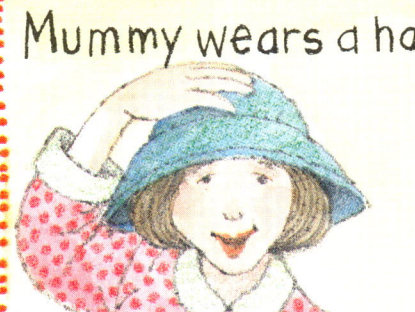
Mummy wears a hat.

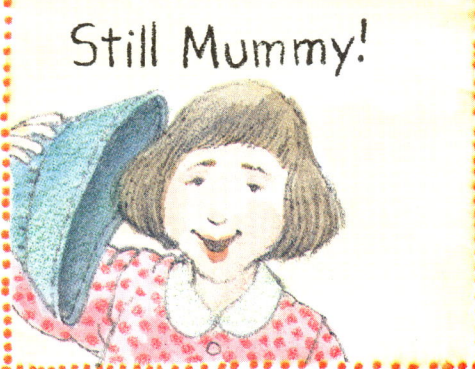
Still Mummy!

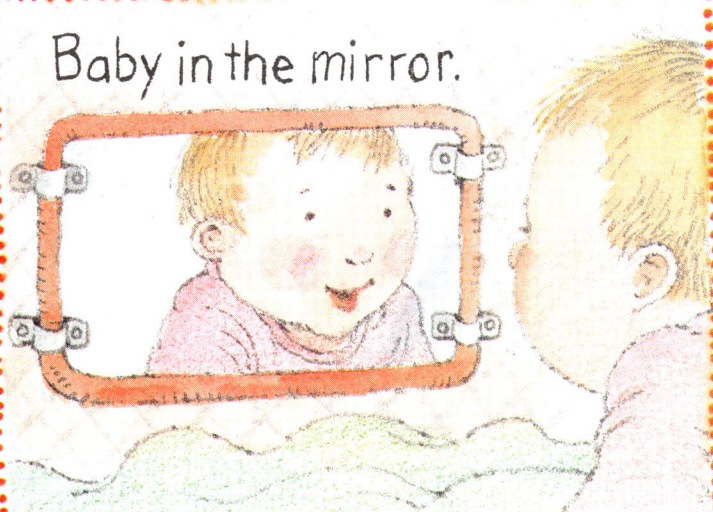
Baby in the mirror.

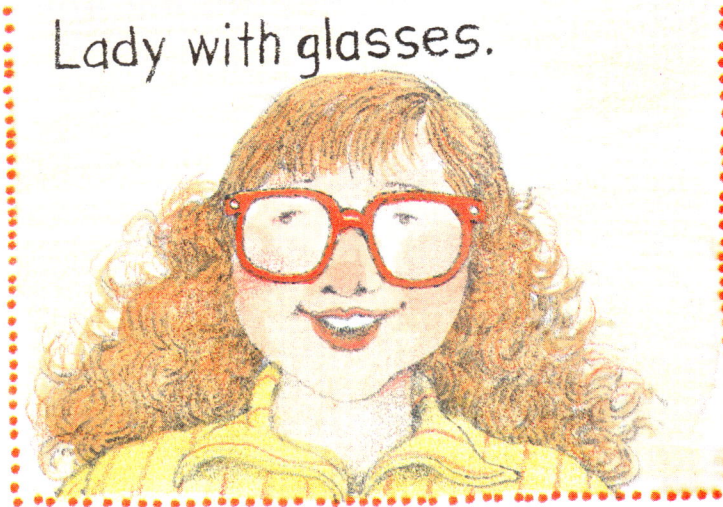
Lady with glasses.

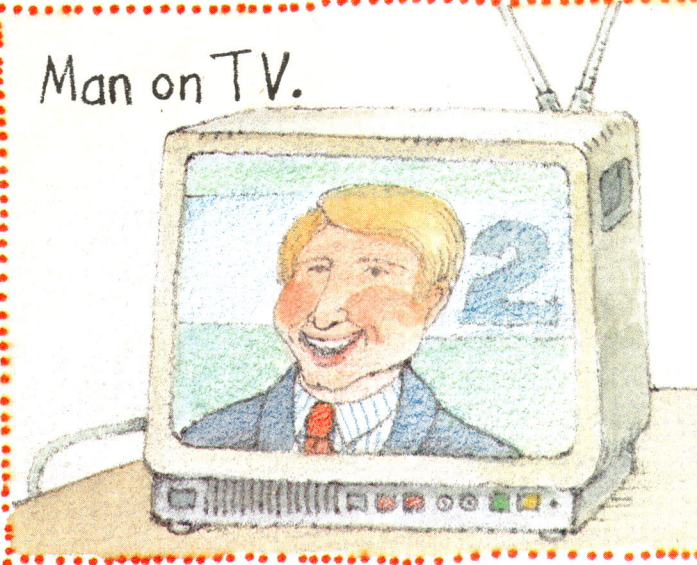
Man on TV.

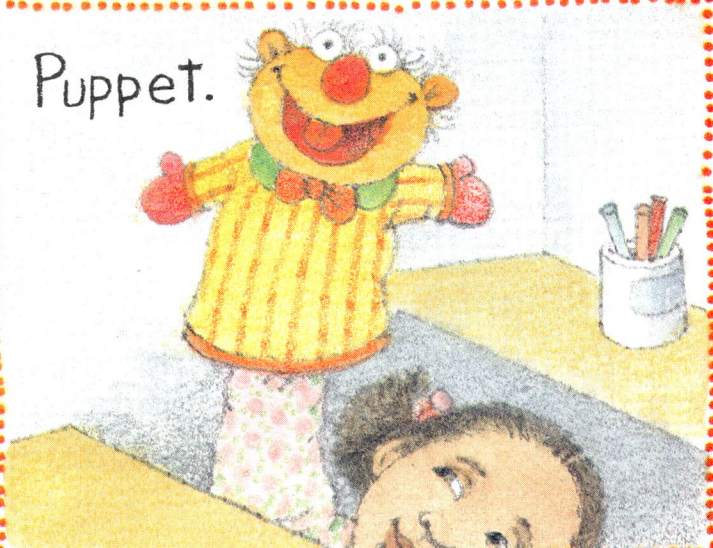
Puppet.

THINGS TO SEE

A baby learns most from things that interest her. Notice what attracts her attention; then tell her its name, talk about it, and, if possible, let her get close to it or handle it.

You can surprise your baby by varying the things you put into a bag or box for her to discover. Use objects that have clear shapes and bright colours.

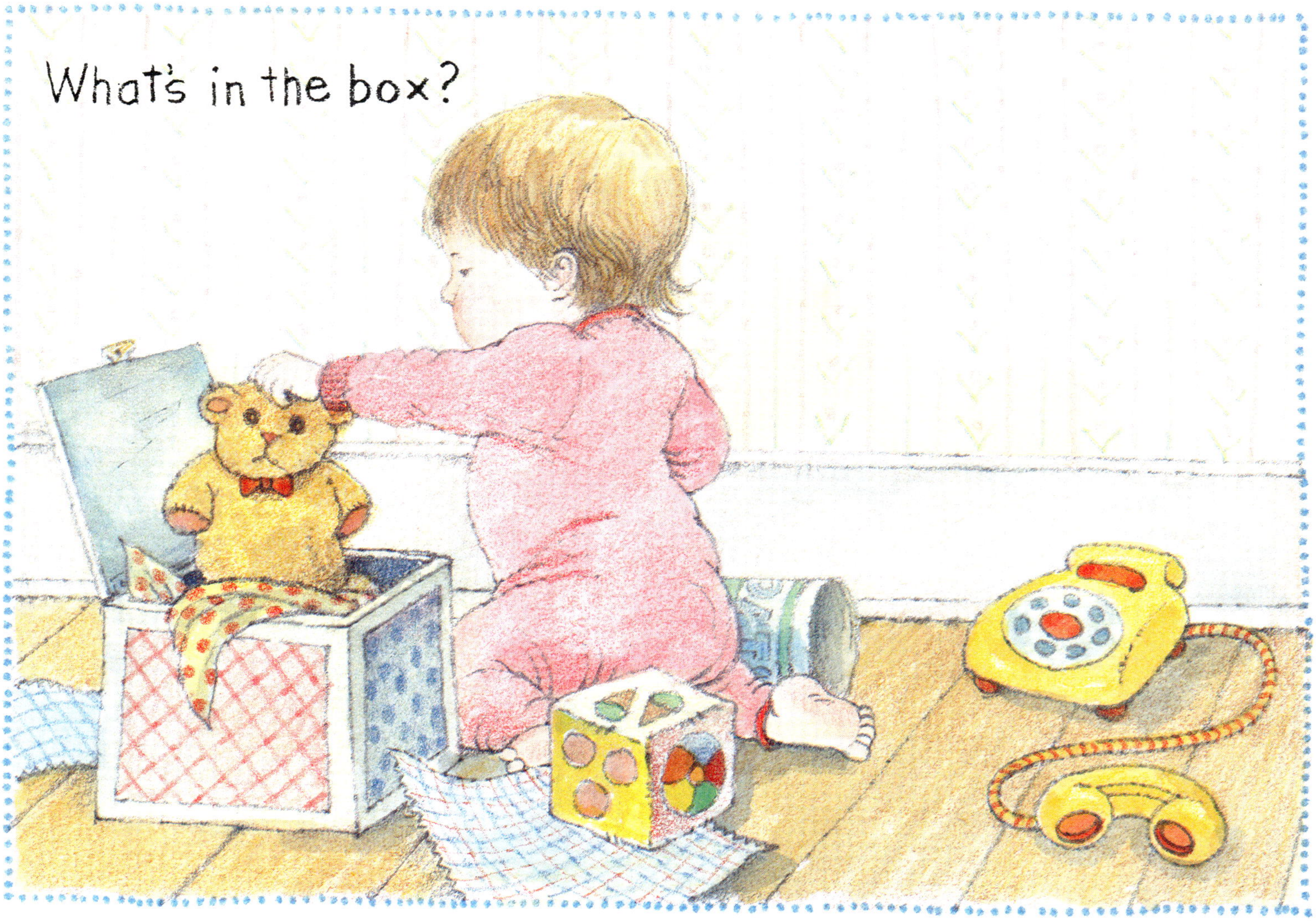

What's in the box?

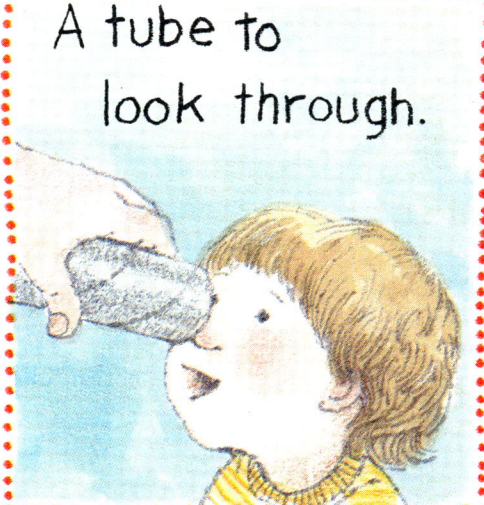

A tube to look through.

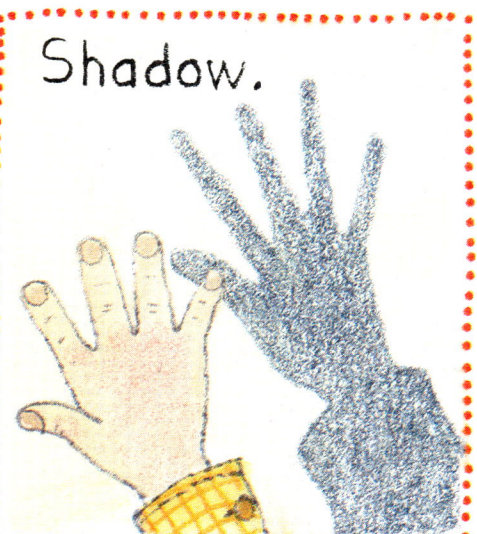

Shadow.

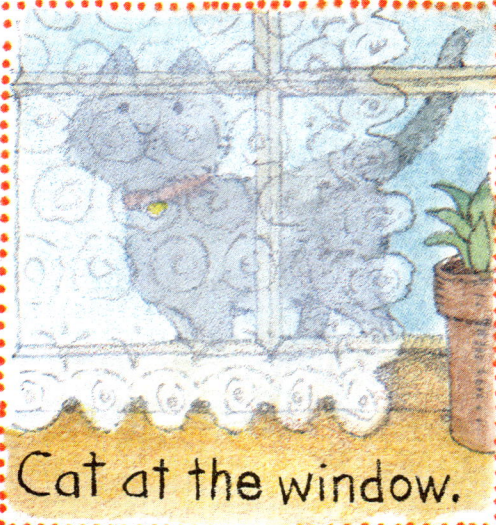

Cat at the window.

PICTURES

Once your baby holds her head up, you can begin showing her pictures. As she gets older, pictures will help her to identify all kinds of things within and beyond her world.

You can use pictures to name something, say what it does, and describe its parts, sounds, size, colour, and anything else that might interest your baby.

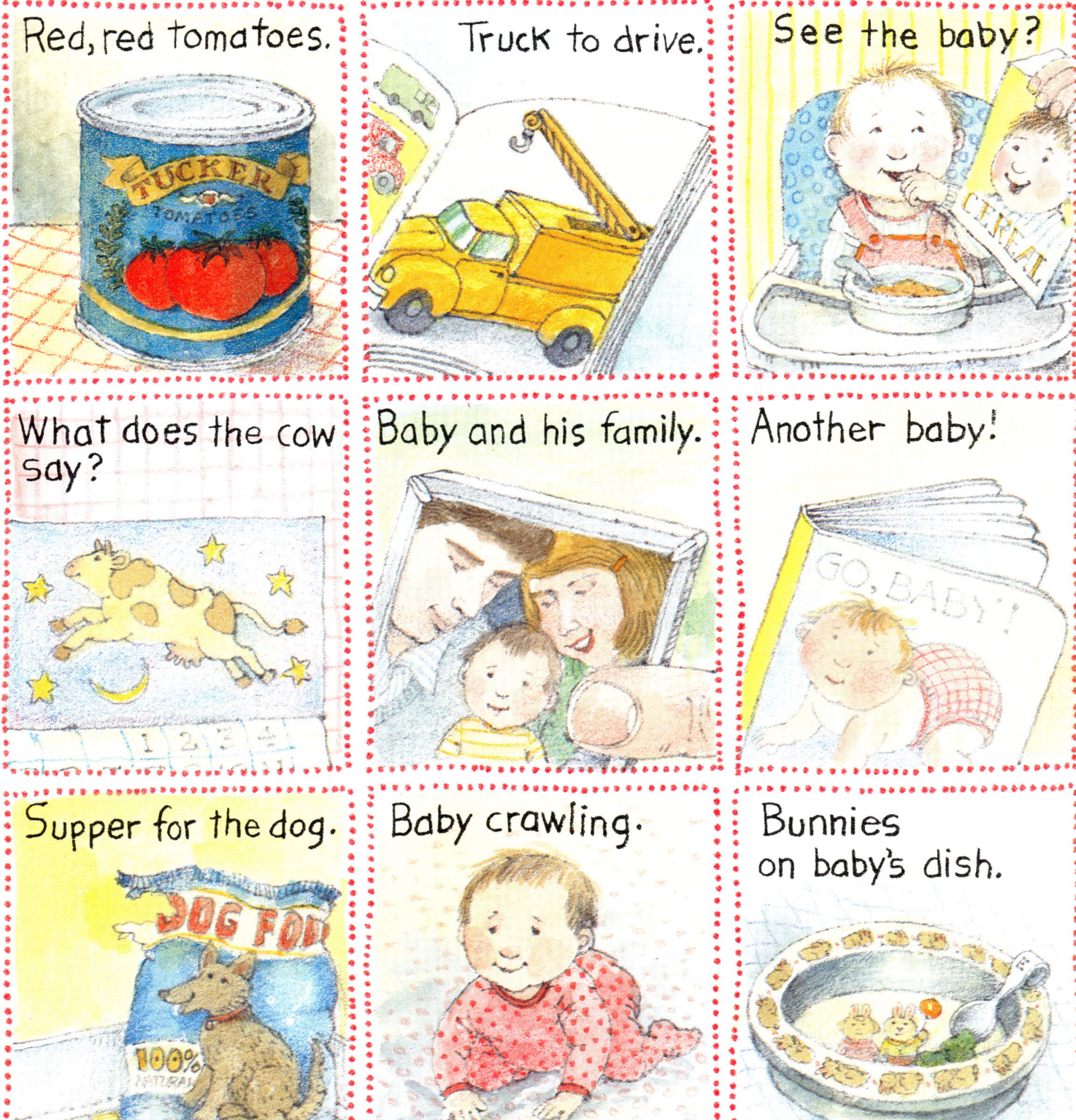

THINGS THAT MOVE

A young baby is more likely to notice an object if it moves. If it has bright colours and makes a noise, all the better. You can interest a baby in many things by moving them and making up sounds for them.

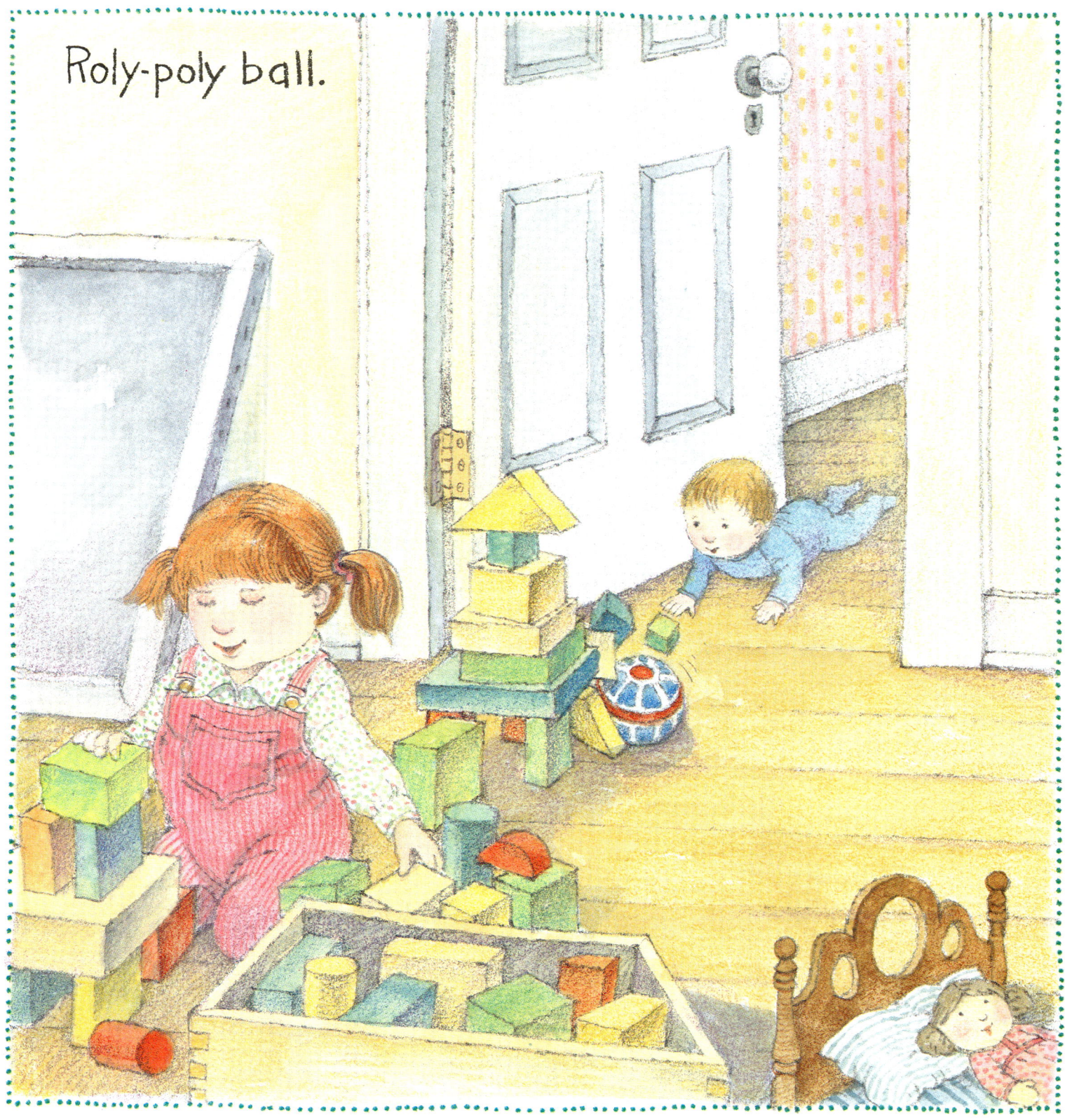

Roly-poly ball.

HOUSEWORK

Let your baby watch you do the housework. Tell her what you're doing, and, as she gets older, let her help. You may appreciate simple tasks in new ways when you see them through your baby's curious eyes.

If your baby is not going to help, have toys or books to hand. A special drawer just for your baby that is filled with toys and safe household gadgets will keep an older baby happily occupied.

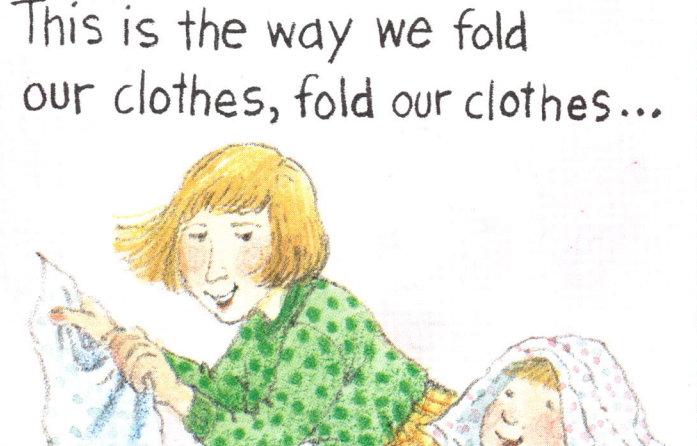

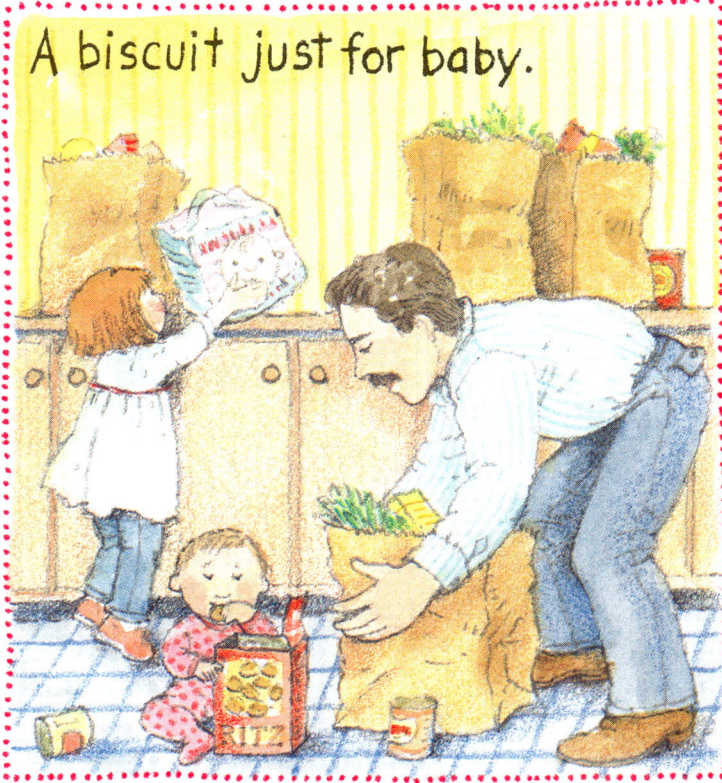

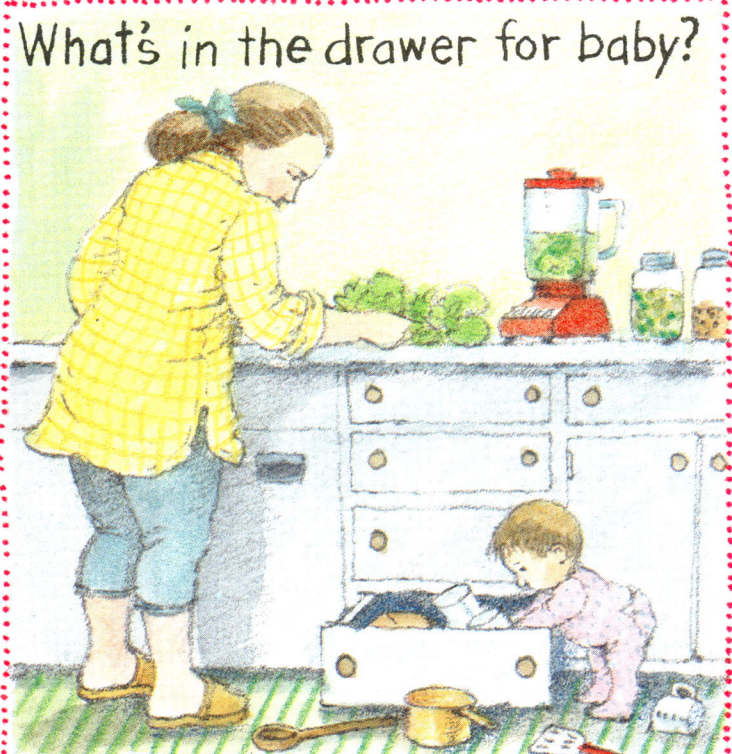

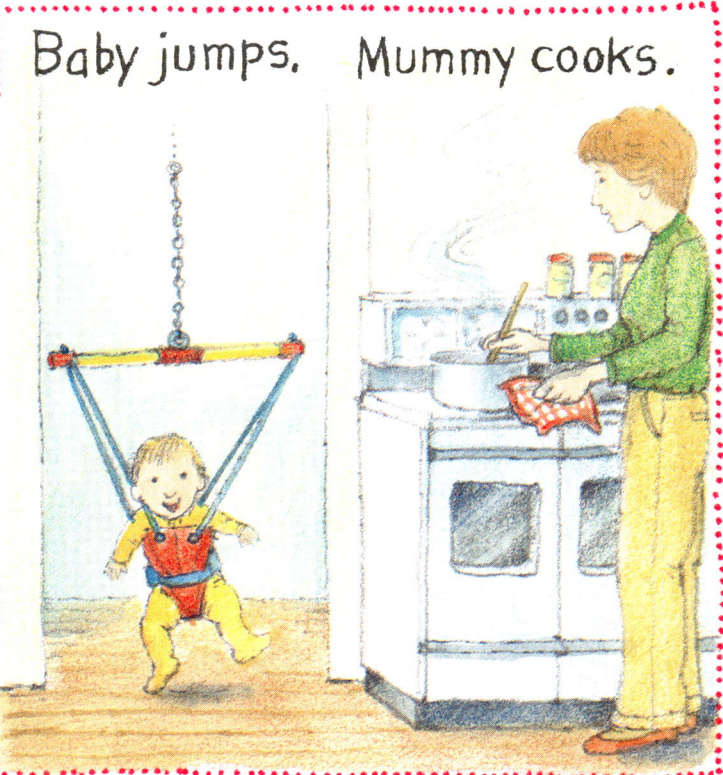

OUT AND ABOUT

Get out in the open with your baby as often as possible. Even a stroll around the block can present endless opportunities to show him the world. Be excited about as many new things as you can; your reaction to something unfamiliar influences how your baby feels about it.

One day your baby will begin pointing out things to you. Then you will see how powerful a little index finger can be.

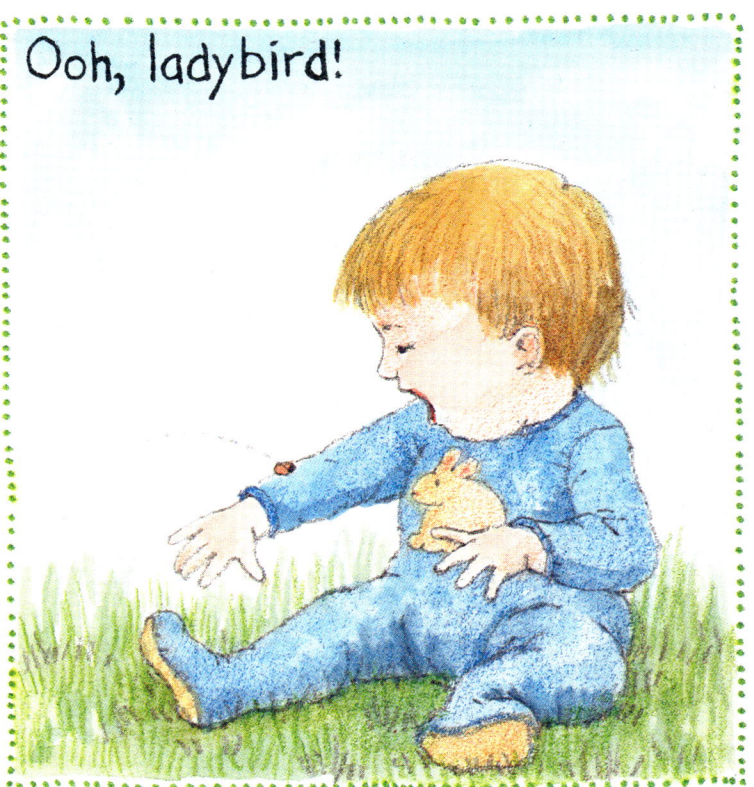

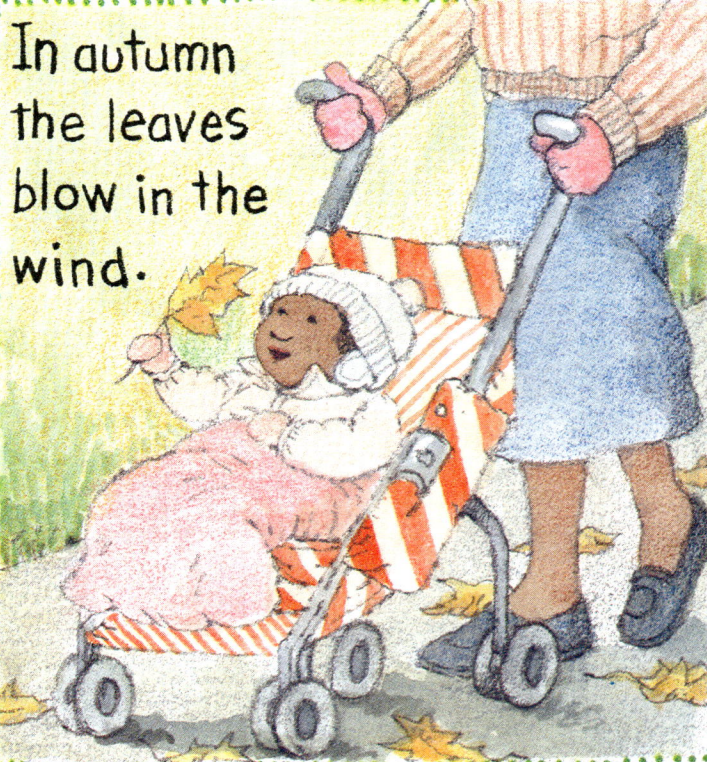

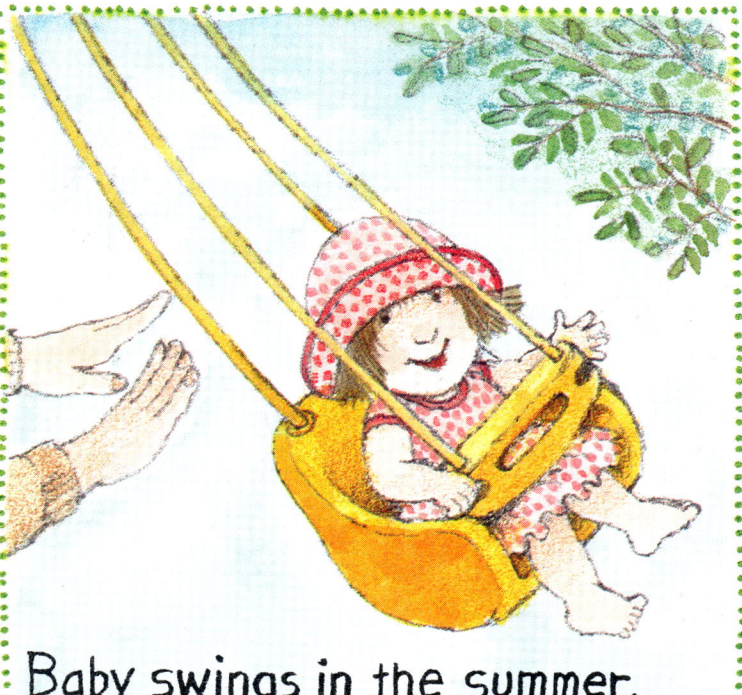

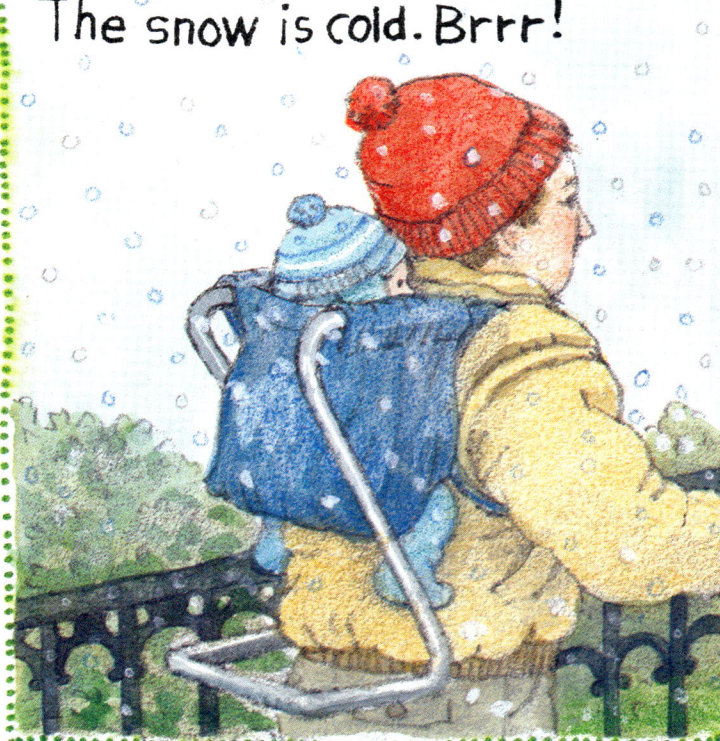

SHOPPING

Shopping is a treat for all the senses. Take advantage of your shopping trips together to point out to your baby all the different things you encounter. Try to find him a little present to enjoy along the way.

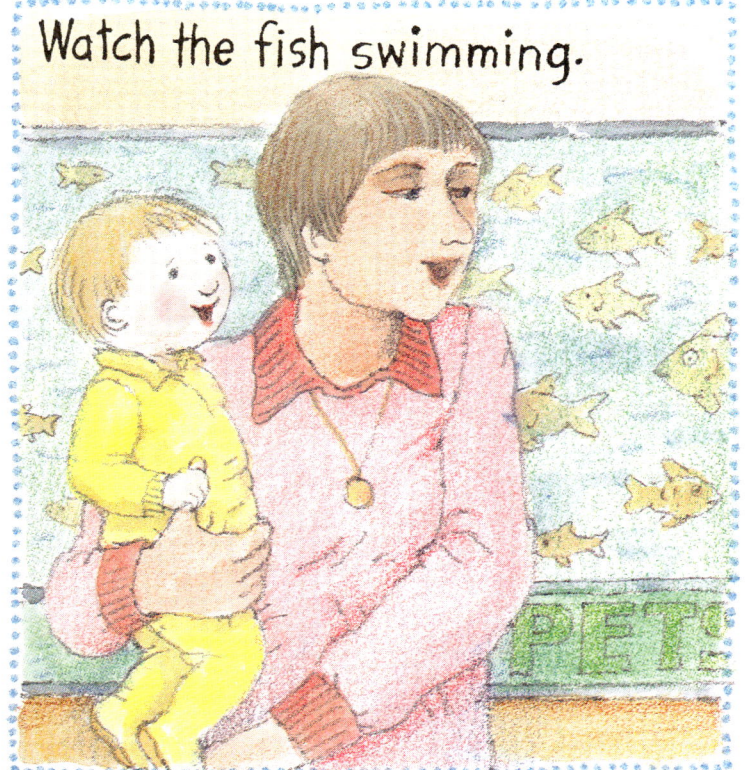
Watch the fish swimming.

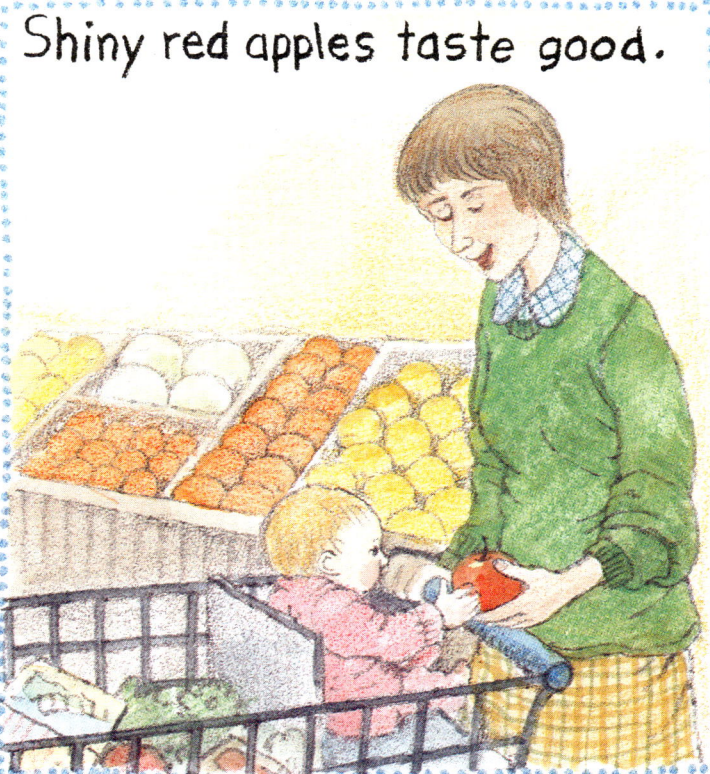
Shiny red apples taste good.

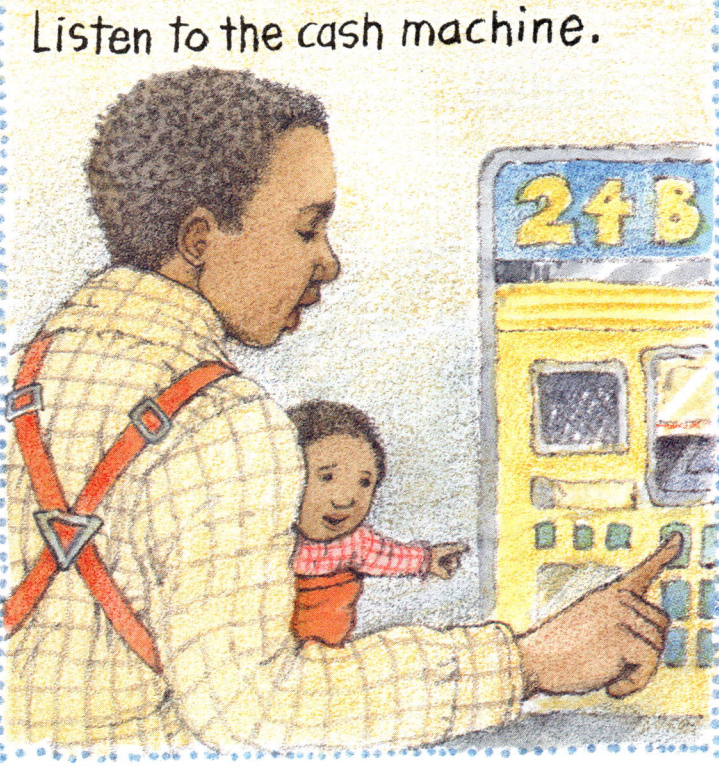
Listen to the cash machine.

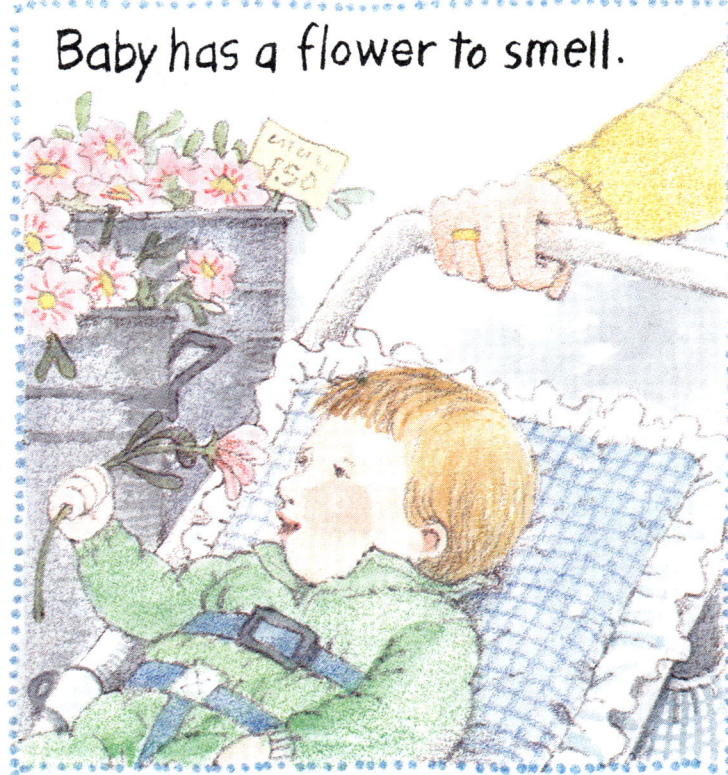
Baby has a flower to smell.

SOUND

No sound interests a new baby more than a human voice. Your young baby will soon follow the sound of your voice with her eyes and listen intently while you speak.

The more you talk to your baby, the more talkative your baby is likely to be. She will practise babbling even when she's alone and enjoy hearing her own voice.

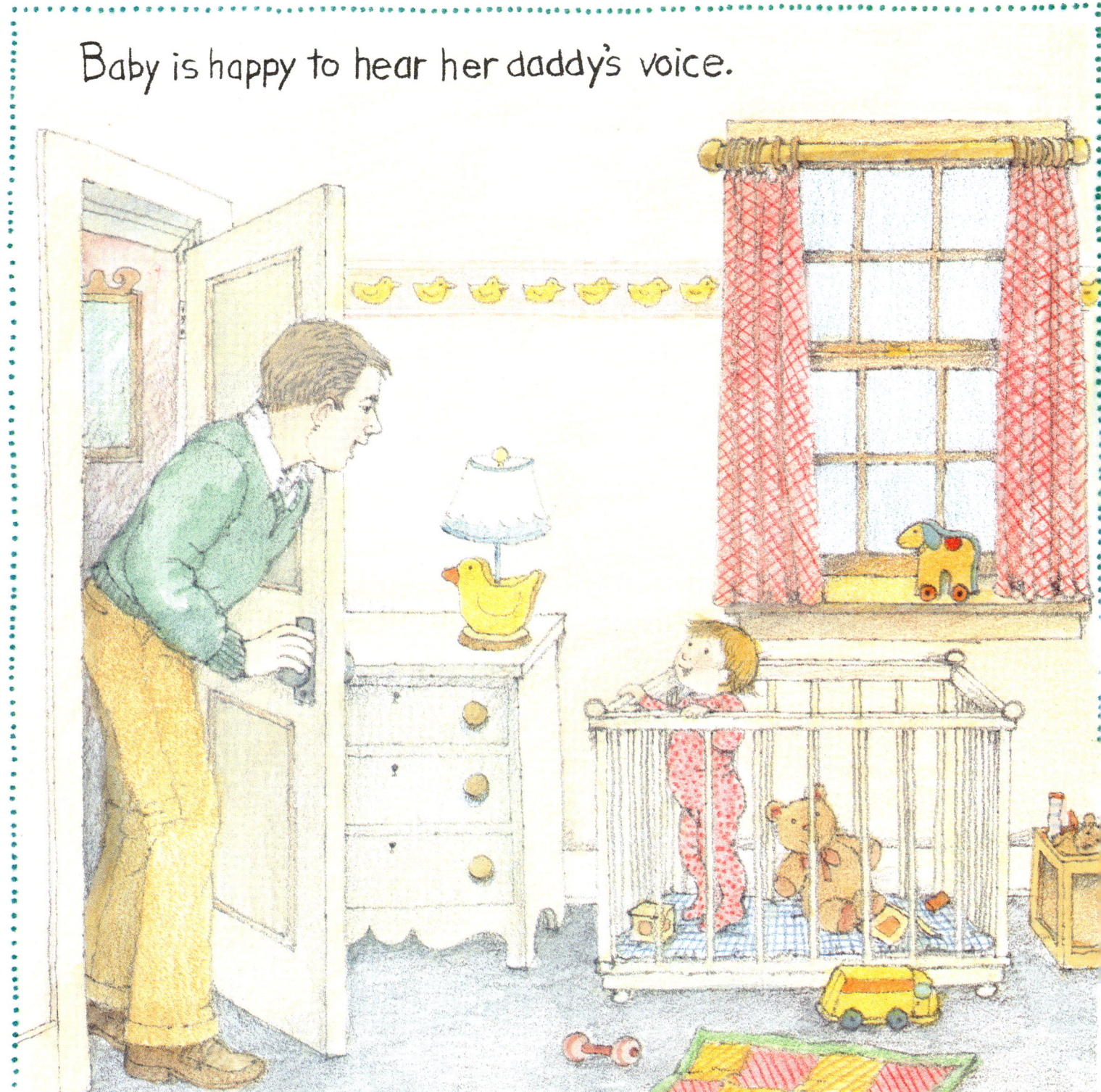

Baby is happy to hear her daddy's voice.

SOUNDS TO HEAR

Help your baby learn about a sound by calling her attention to it, imitating it, and naming its source.

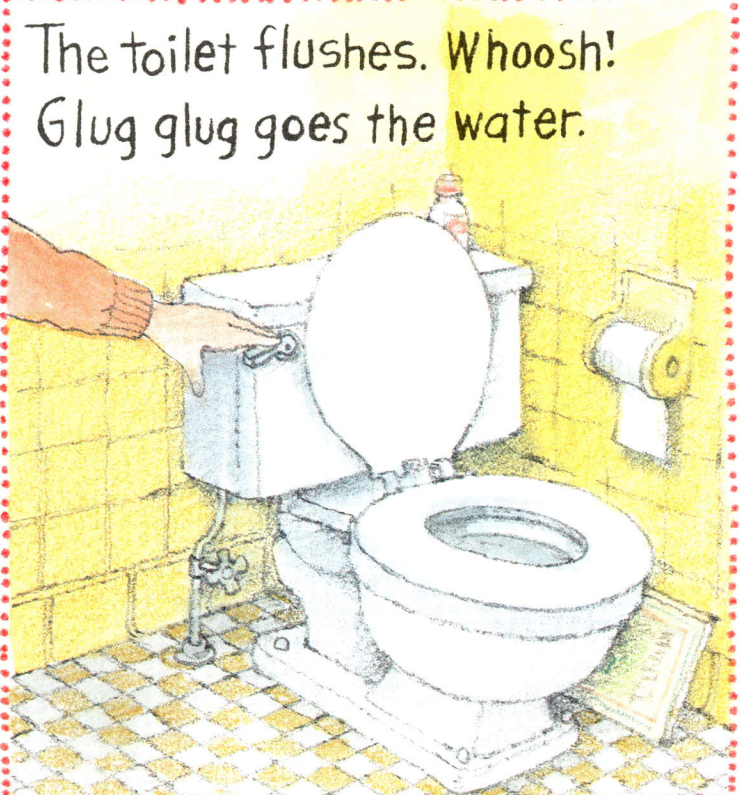

The toilet flushes. Whoosh! Glug glug goes the water.

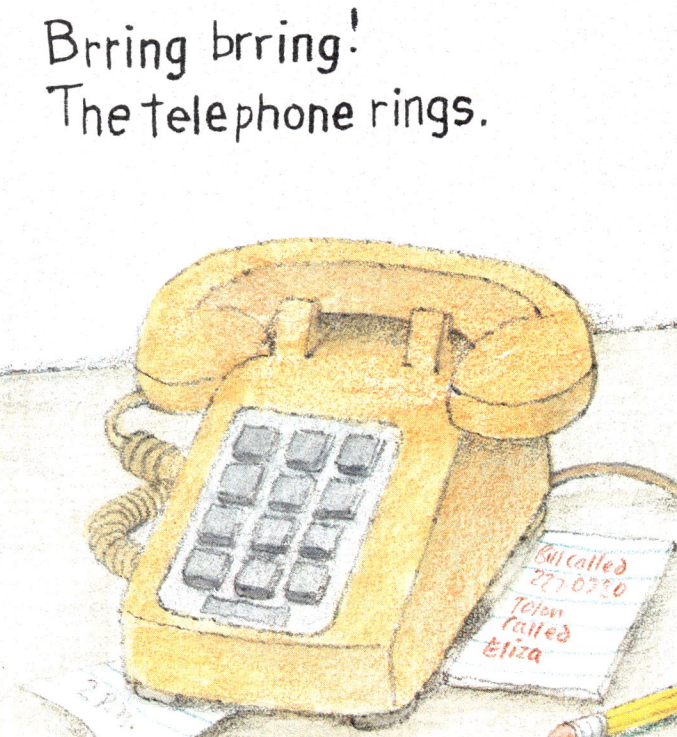

Brring brring! The telephone rings.

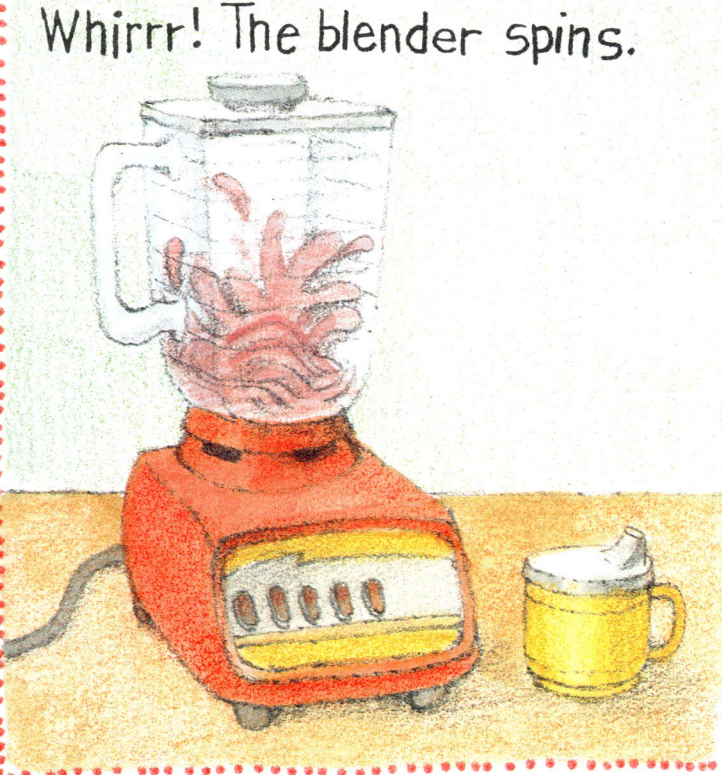

Whirrr! The blender spins.

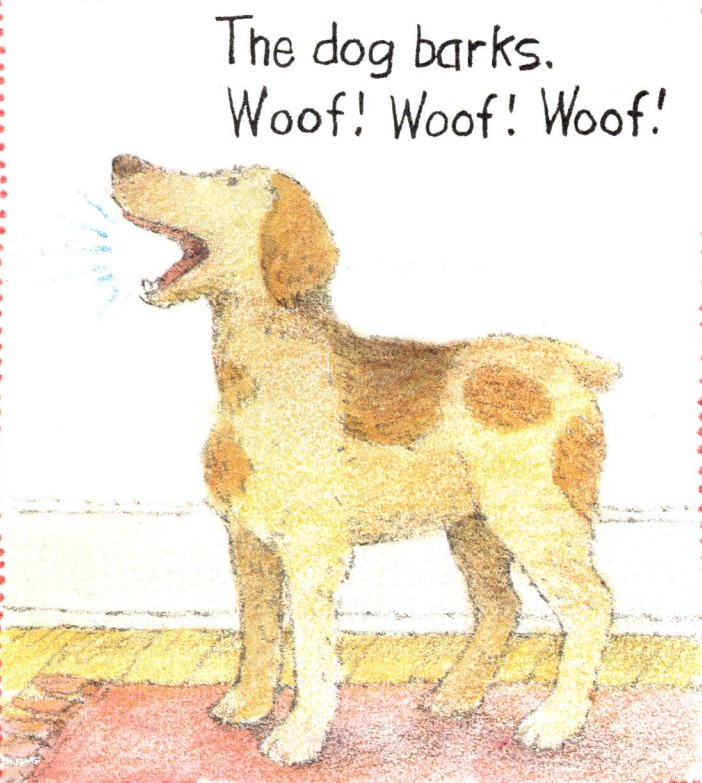

The dog barks. Woof! Woof! Woof!

SOUNDS TO MAKE

Once your baby can hold on to things with his hands, he will love making noises with them. Encourage him to produce all kinds of sounds.

Invent rattles by filling safe containers with dried beans, buttons, bells, and coins.

Everyday things you may take for granted will delight your baby as toys.

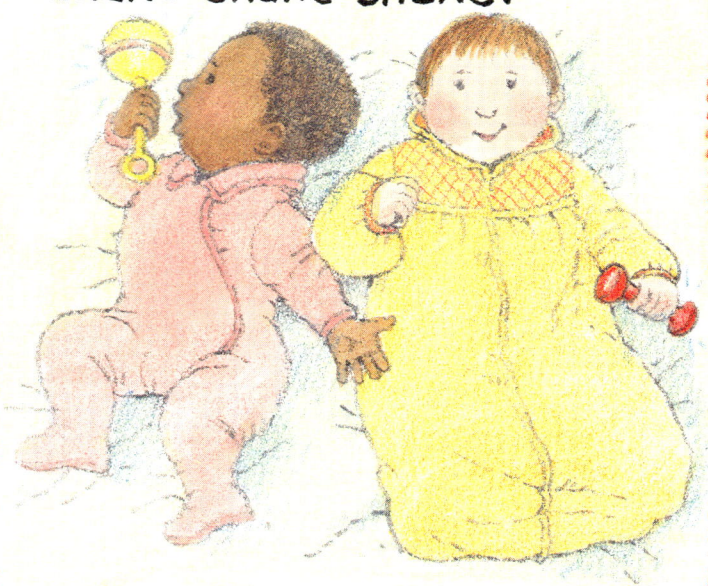
Babies shake their rattles. Shake shake shake!

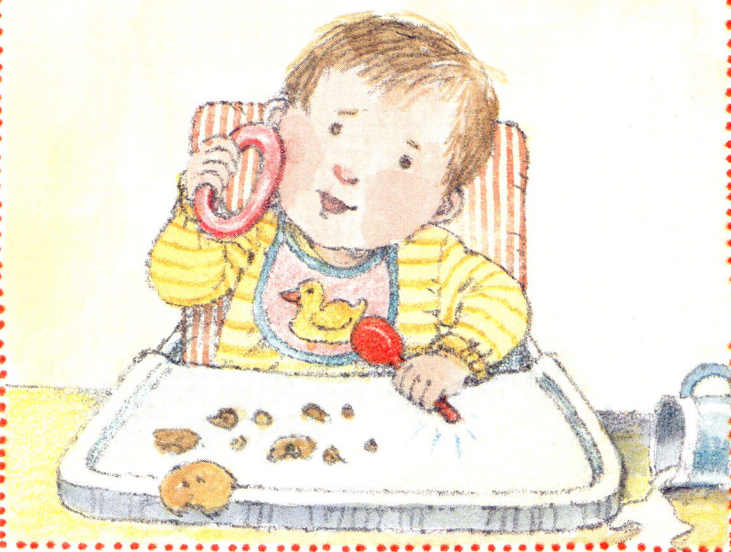
Baby bang bang banging on his tray.

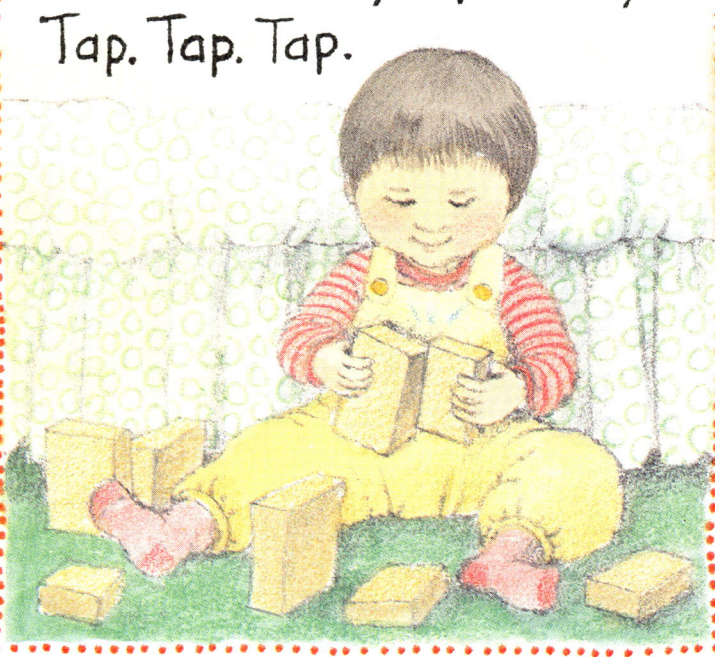
Shhh. Now baby taps softly. Tap. Tap. Tap.

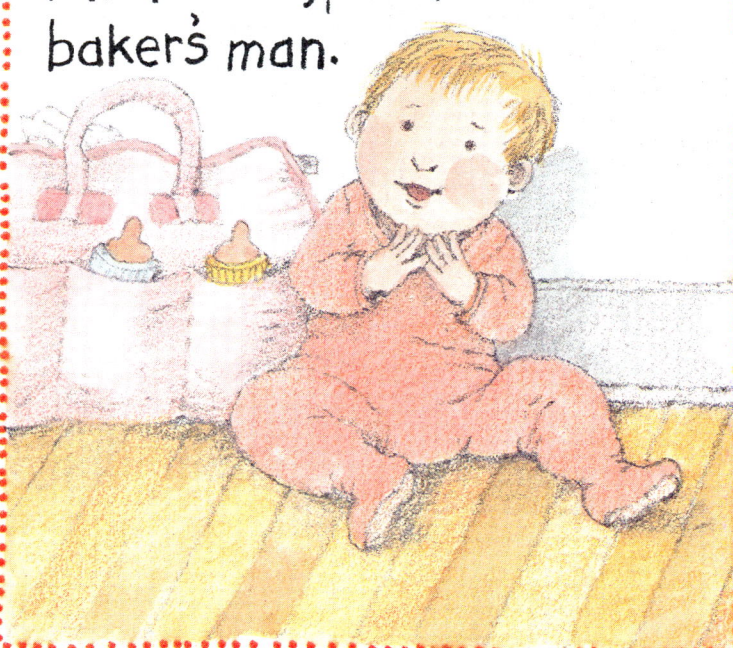
Pat-a-cake, pat-a-cake, baker's man.

CONVERSATION

Good conversation requires listening as well as speaking. Comment on things your baby sees or does, and give him time to respond in his own way. Try repeating the sounds he makes. Then he'll know you've been listening.

Call your baby by name. It will help both of you to learn that he's a person in his own right.

Tape-record your baby's voice from time to time and play it back. You'll appreciate his progress. Remember to save the tape for him!

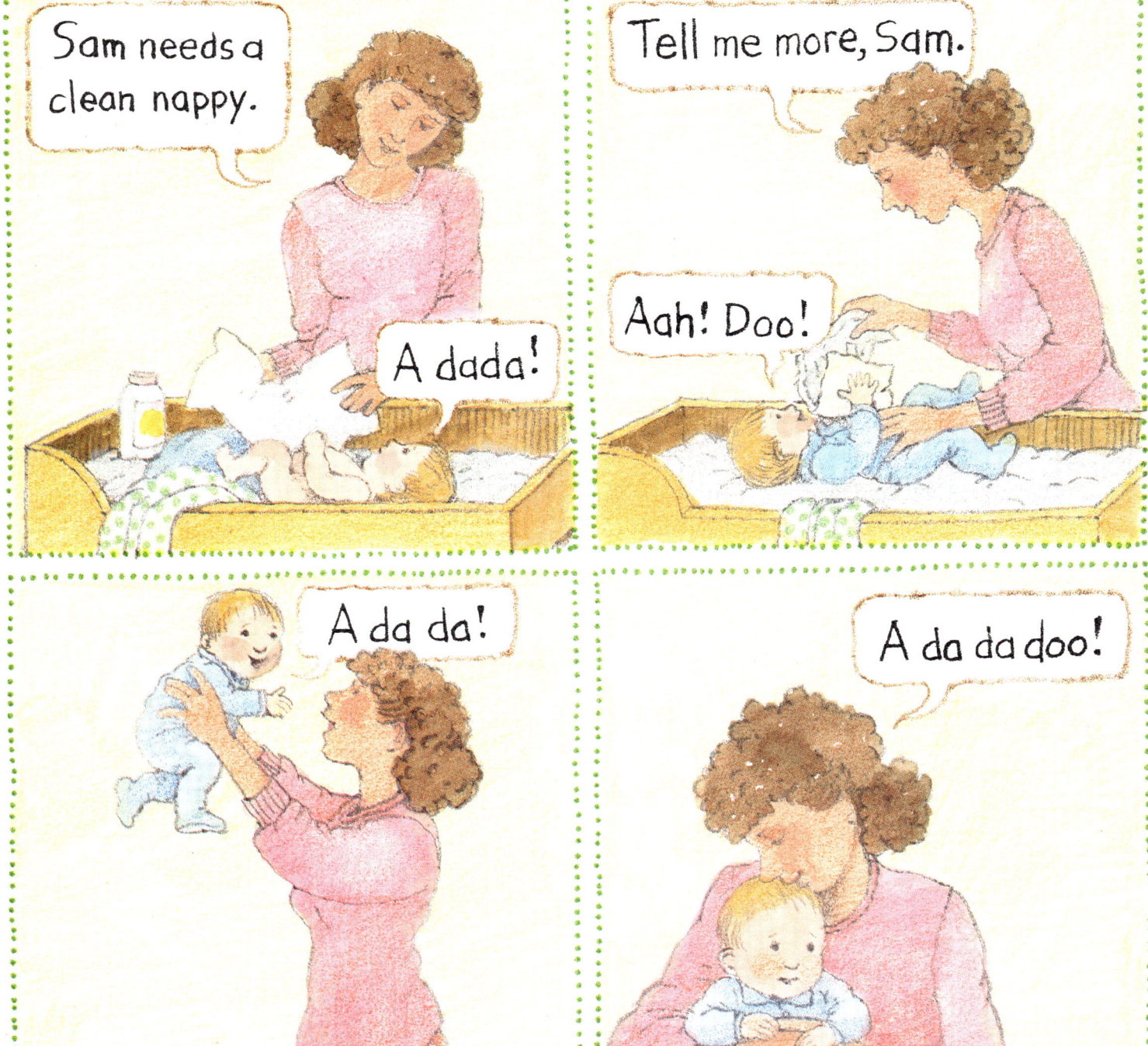

TONE OF VOICE

How you speak to a baby is more important than *what* you say. Your tone of voice shows your feelings and can influence your baby's behaviour. A shouting voice often upsets a calm baby, but a soft, gentle voice can calm an upset baby.

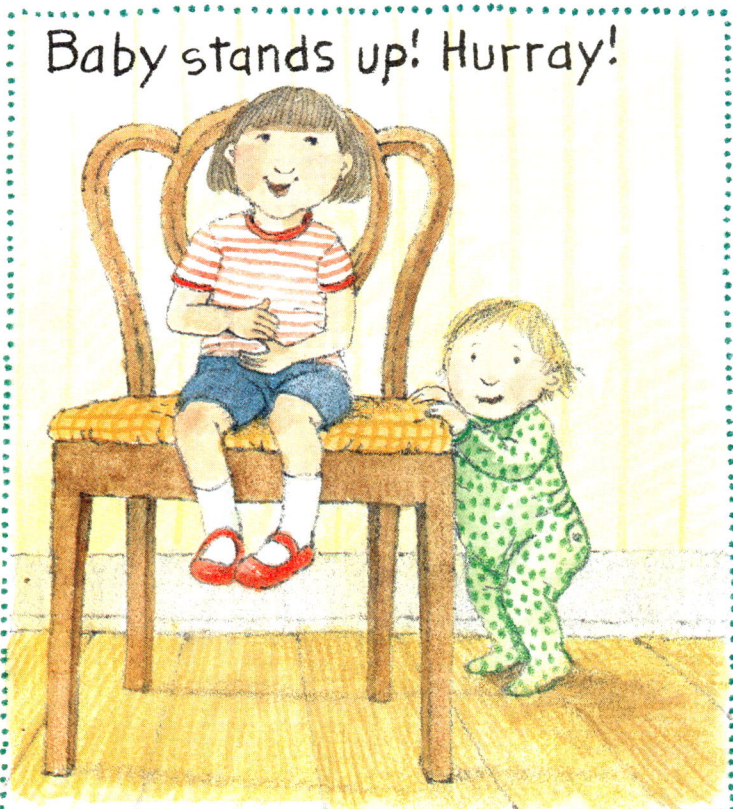

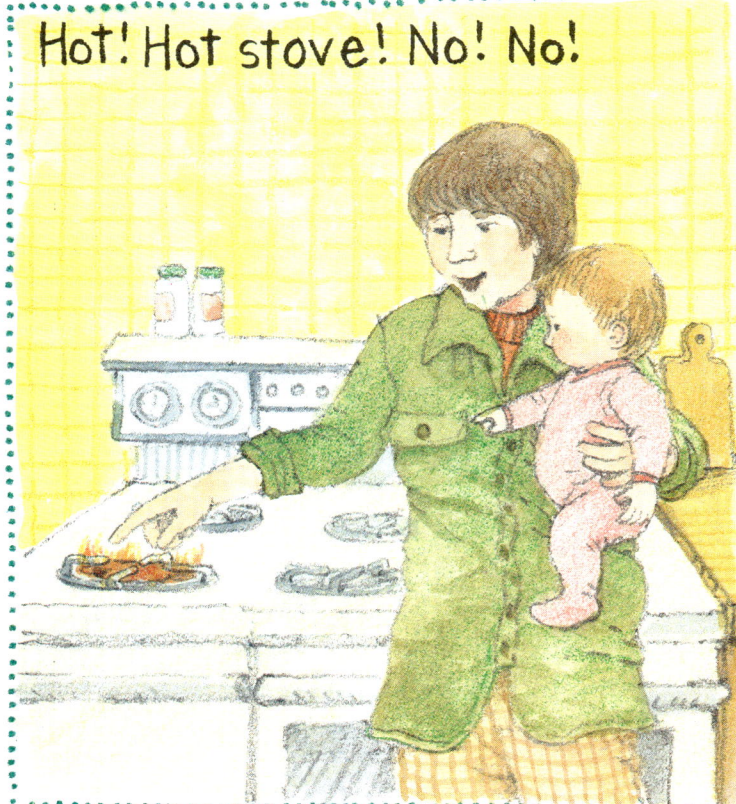

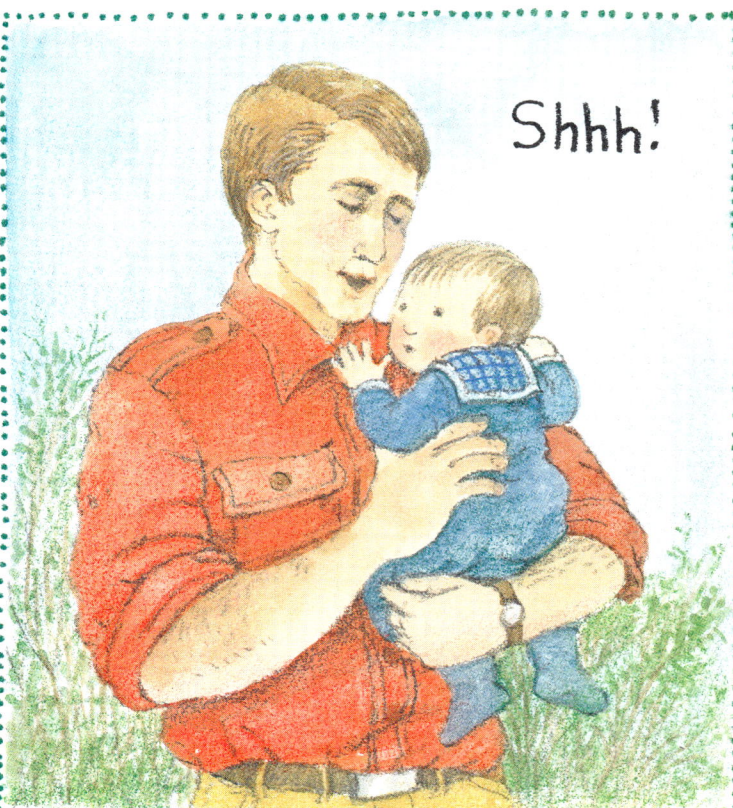

GESTURES SPEAK TOO

Babies can express themselves long before they learn to talk. They communicate with you using facial expressions, gestures, and sounds. Sometimes you have to "listen" with your eyes!

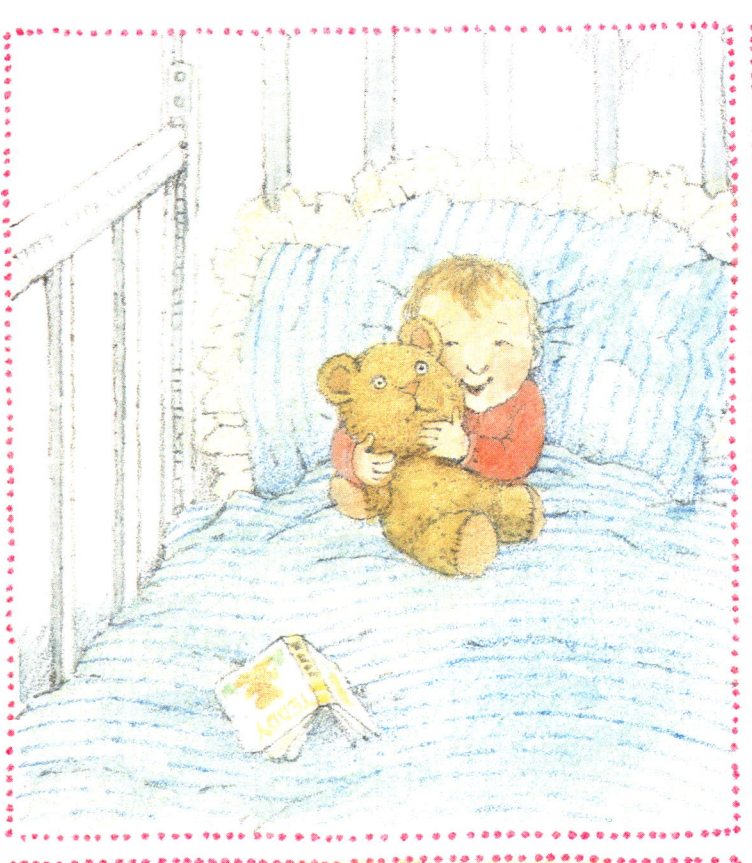
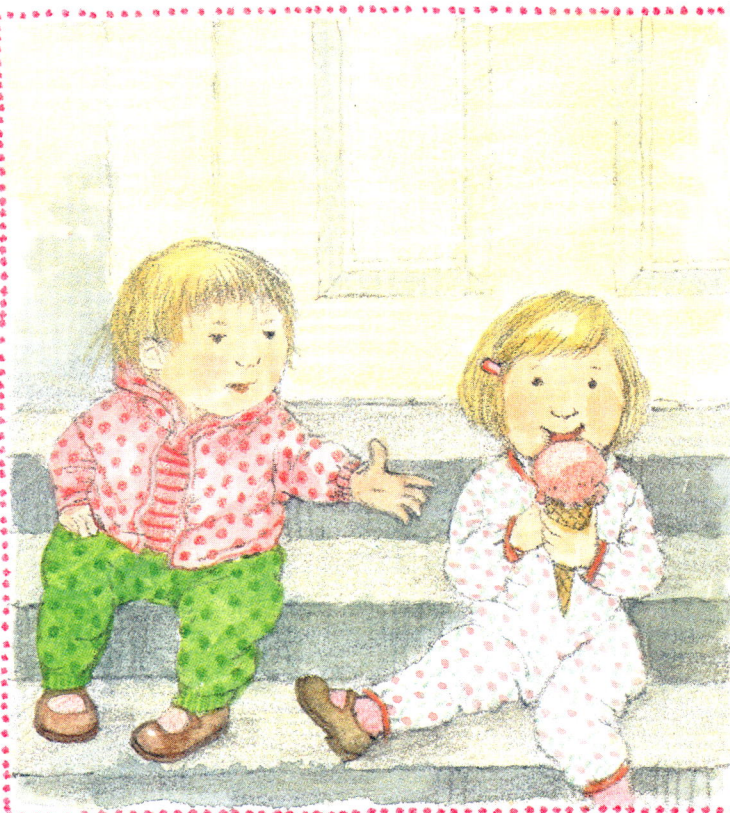
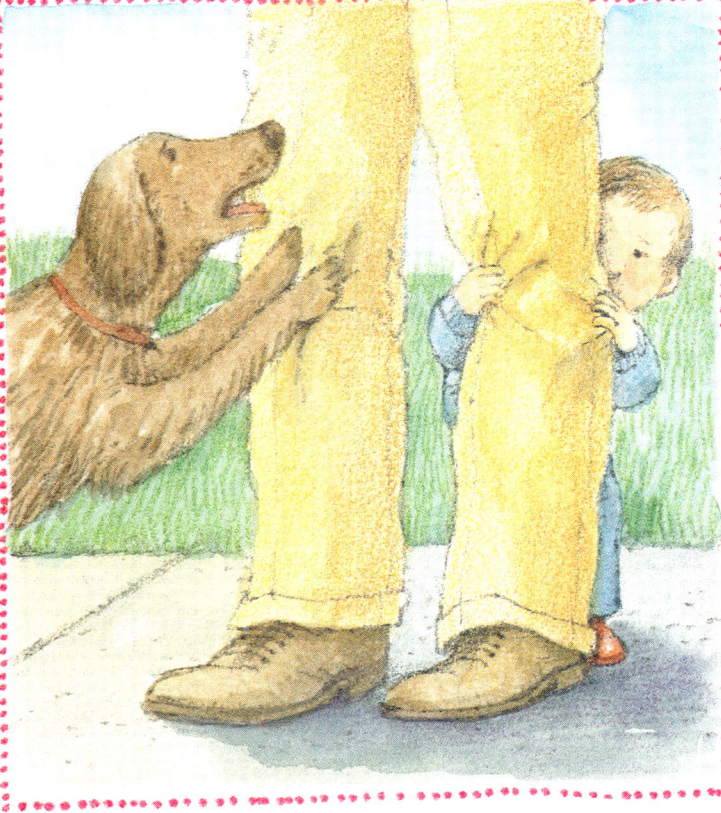
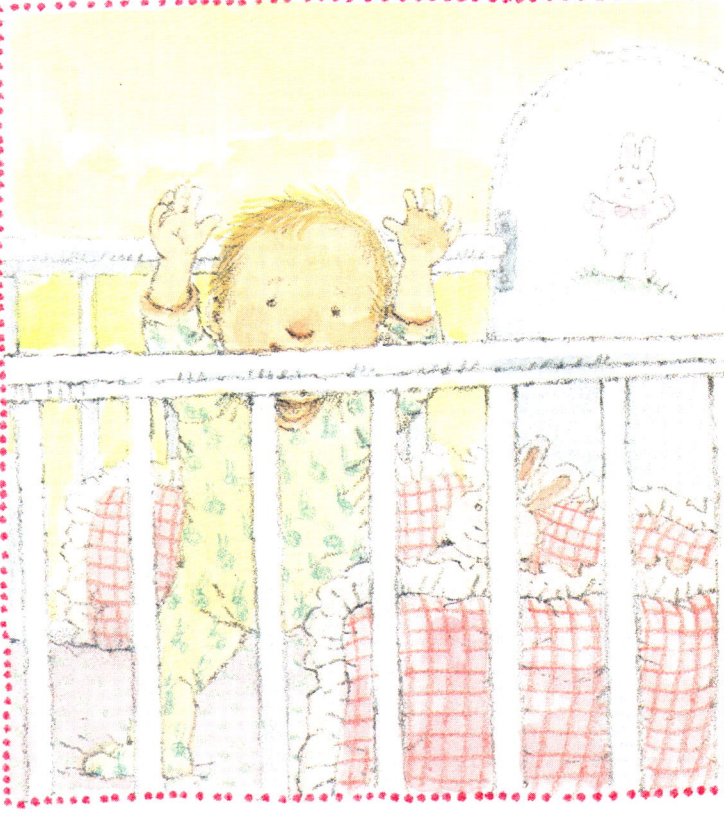

READING AND RHYMING

Get into the habit of reading books and magazines to your baby every day. This will foster a love for books and an eagerness to learn to read later on. Remember reading to your baby can mean just pointing out the pictures on the page.

Fit rhymes into your everyday routines whenever you can. Listening to rhymes helps develop your baby's language skills. Make sure you have a good selection of nursery rhyme books. Have fun thinking up nonsense words to rhyme and repeat.

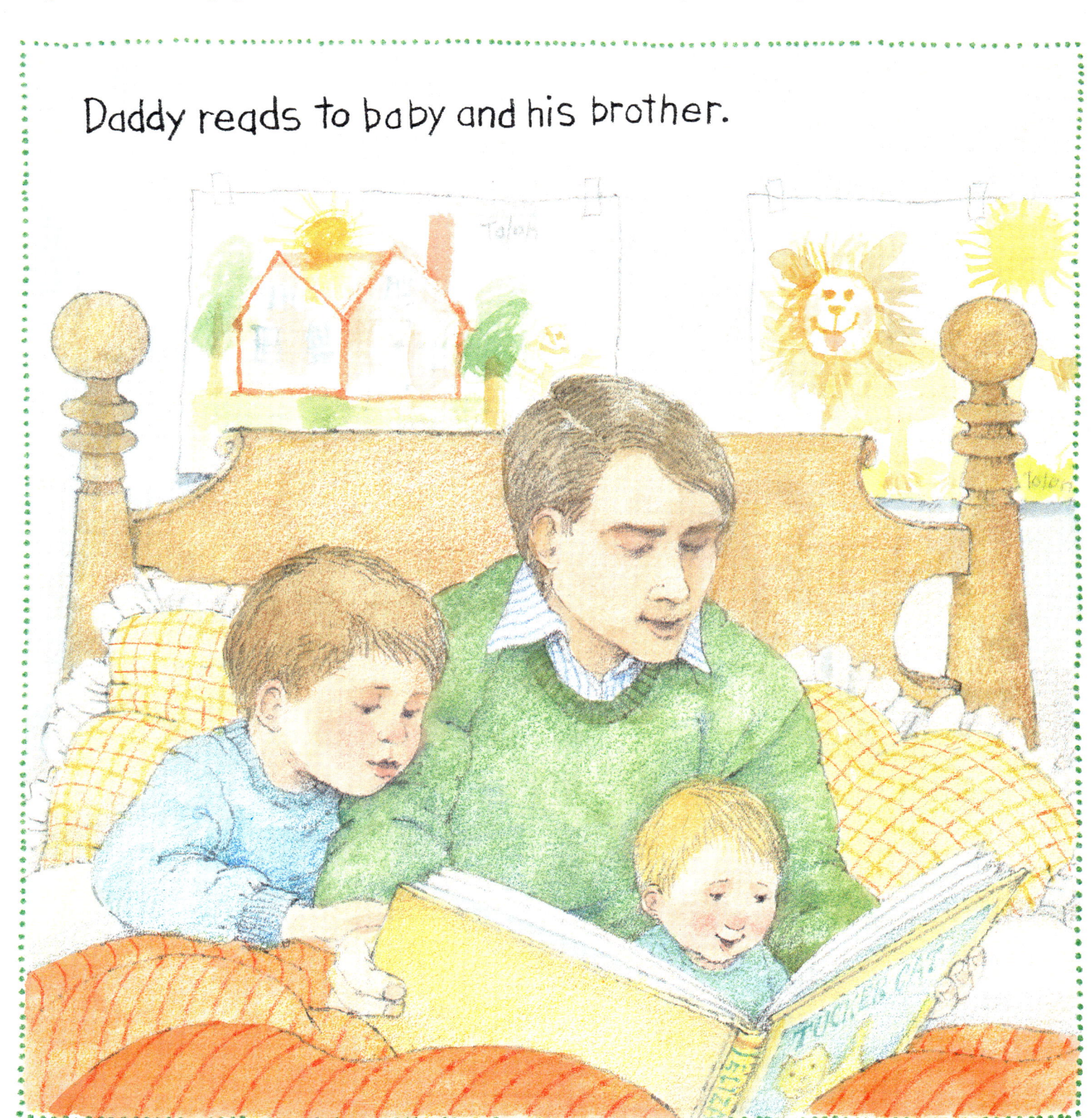

Daddy reads to baby and his brother.

MUSIC AND DANCE

Babies are never too young to be introduced to music and dance. They like tunes with a simple beat and clear melody. Try singing along, clapping, or moving your baby's body to the beat. Play recordings of nursery rhymes and children's songs. Take tapes along on car journeys. Let your baby hear live music at a parade or outdoor concert.

Sing to your baby. The simplest, silliest tunes will please her, especially if you sing them. Treat her to a lullaby at bedtime.

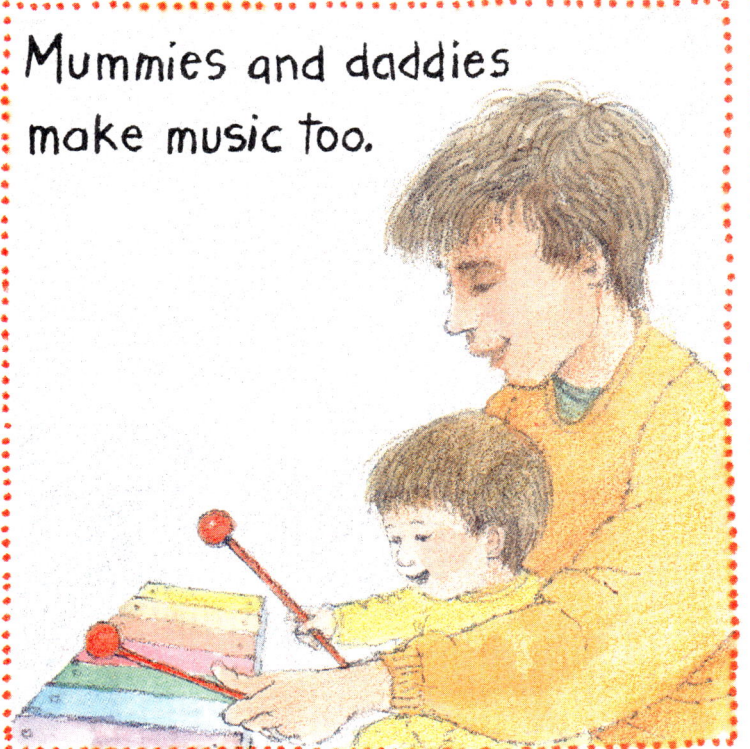

Mummies and daddies make music too.

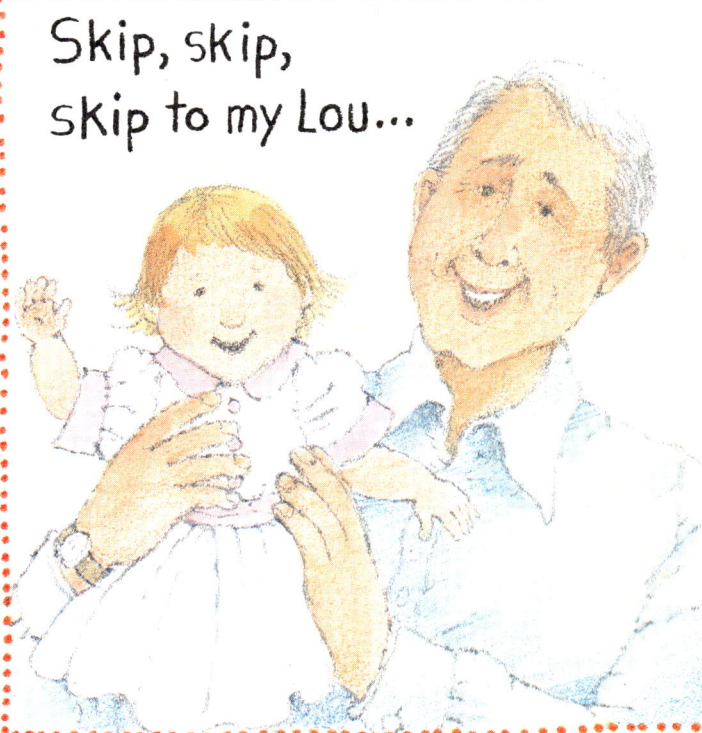

Skip, skip, skip to my Lou...

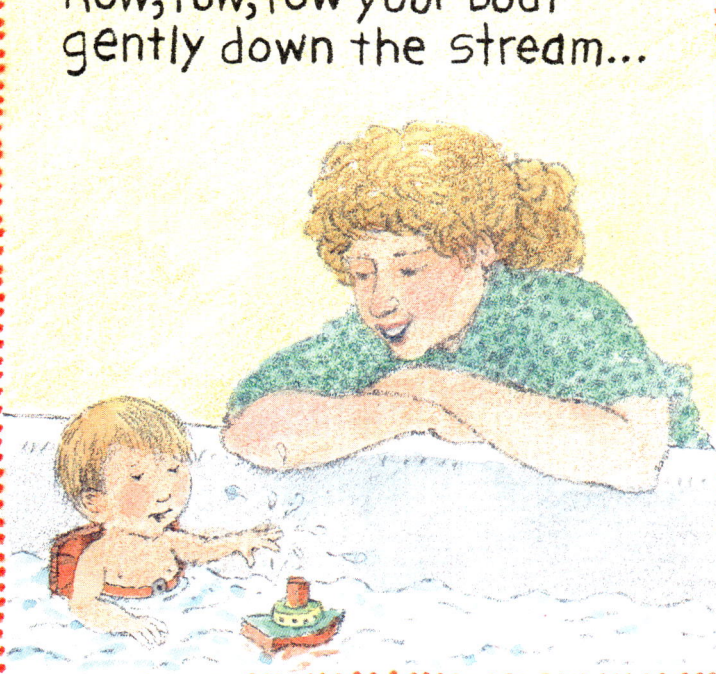

Row, row, row your boat gently down the stream...

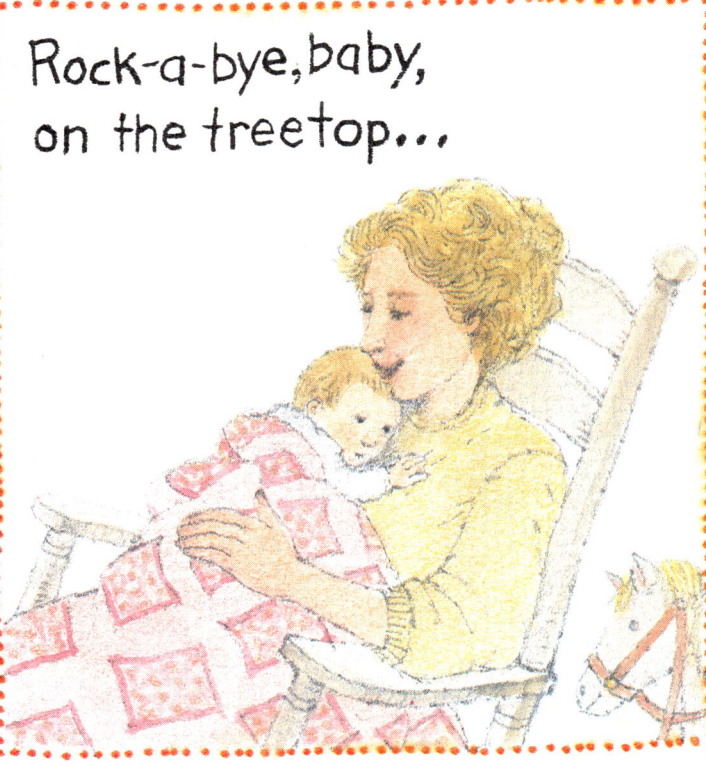

Rock-a-bye, baby, on the treetop...

TASTE AND SMELL

Feeding is a baby's first and most important experience of taste and smell, two closely related senses. A baby's feeding also satisfies much more than hunger: by being fed on time and given enough time to suck, by being held, smiled at, and enjoyed, a baby learns to trust the people in his world.

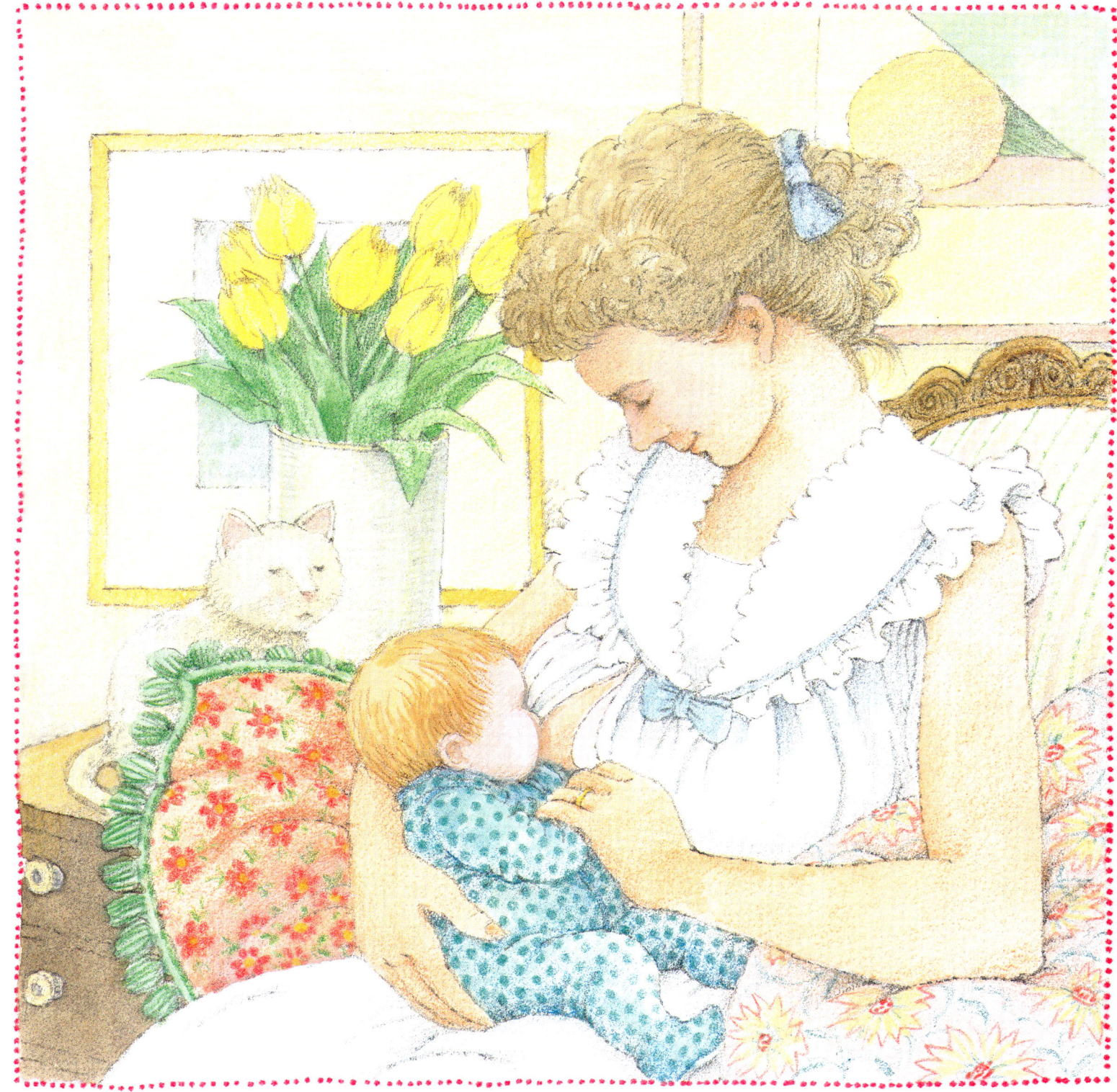

THINGS TO SMELL

Help your baby to enjoy fragrant things by showing her how to smell. She may want to taste good-smelling things whether or not they are edible, so be prepared to act quickly!

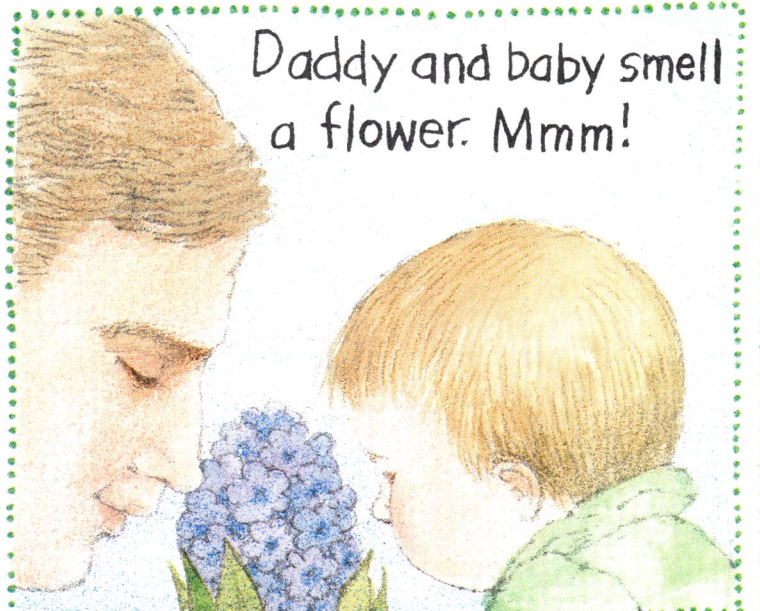
Daddy and baby smell a flower. Mmm!

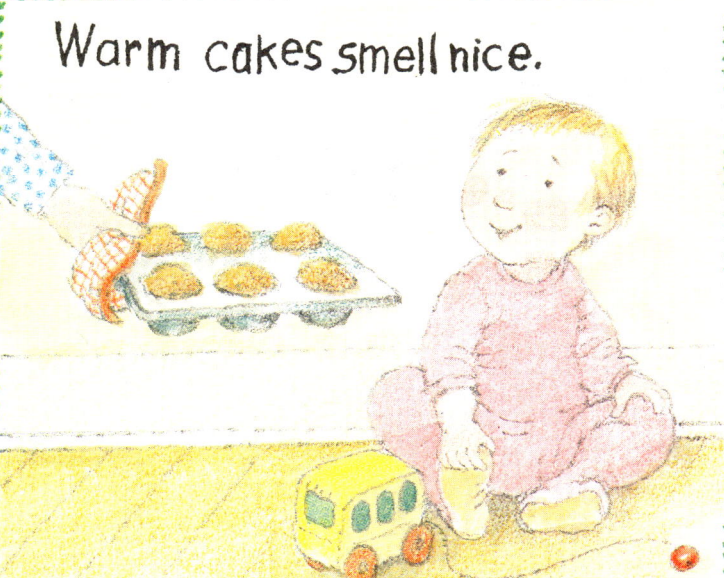
Warm cakes smell nice.

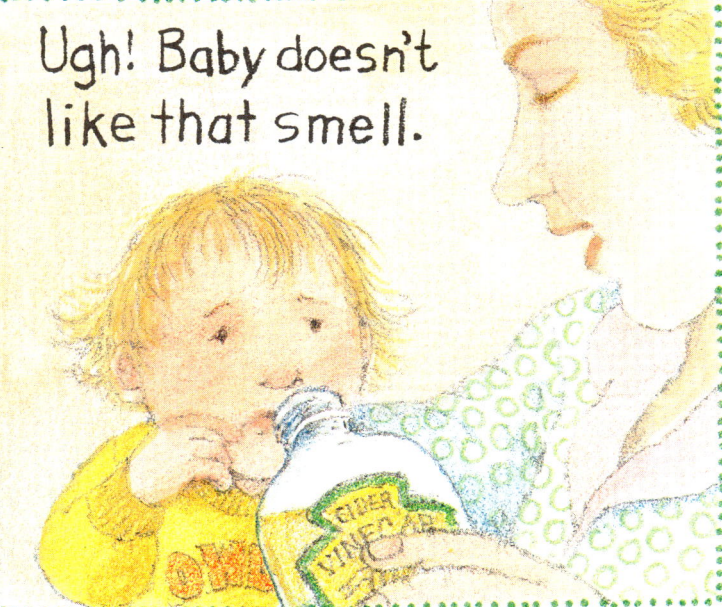
Ugh! Baby doesn't like that smell.

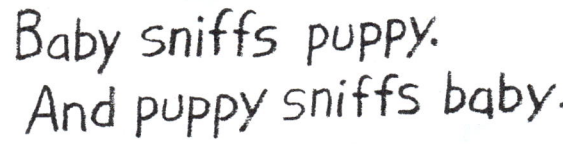
Baby sniffs puppy. And puppy sniffs baby.

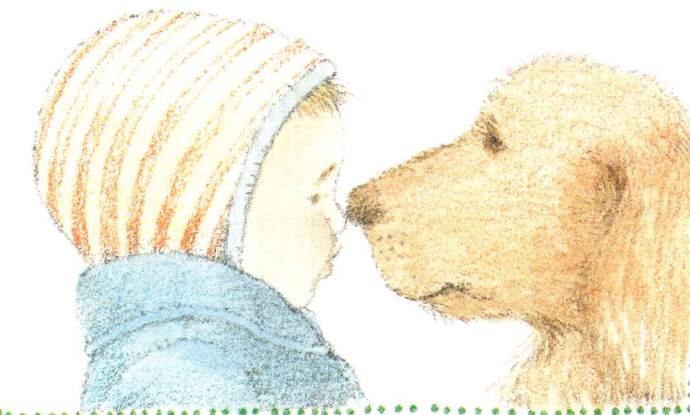

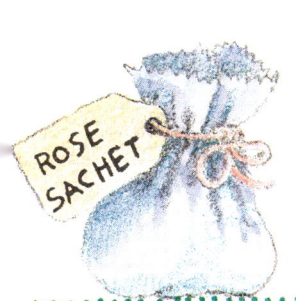 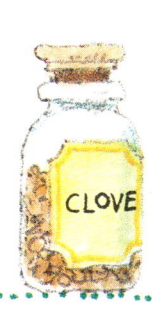 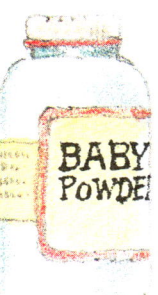  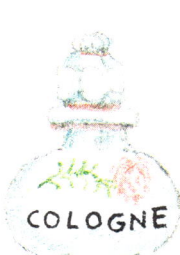 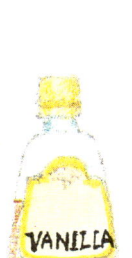 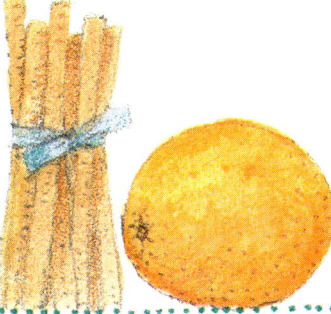

EATING

Give an older baby balanced meals and let him taste and smell many different foods. Introduce new dishes one at a time. Be excited about meals and show your baby that you will try what you feed him. Don't try to force him to eat a food; instead, try it another time and perhaps in another form. Your baby can feed himself with his fingers while you help with a spoon. Later he can practise getting a small spoon to his mouth by himself.

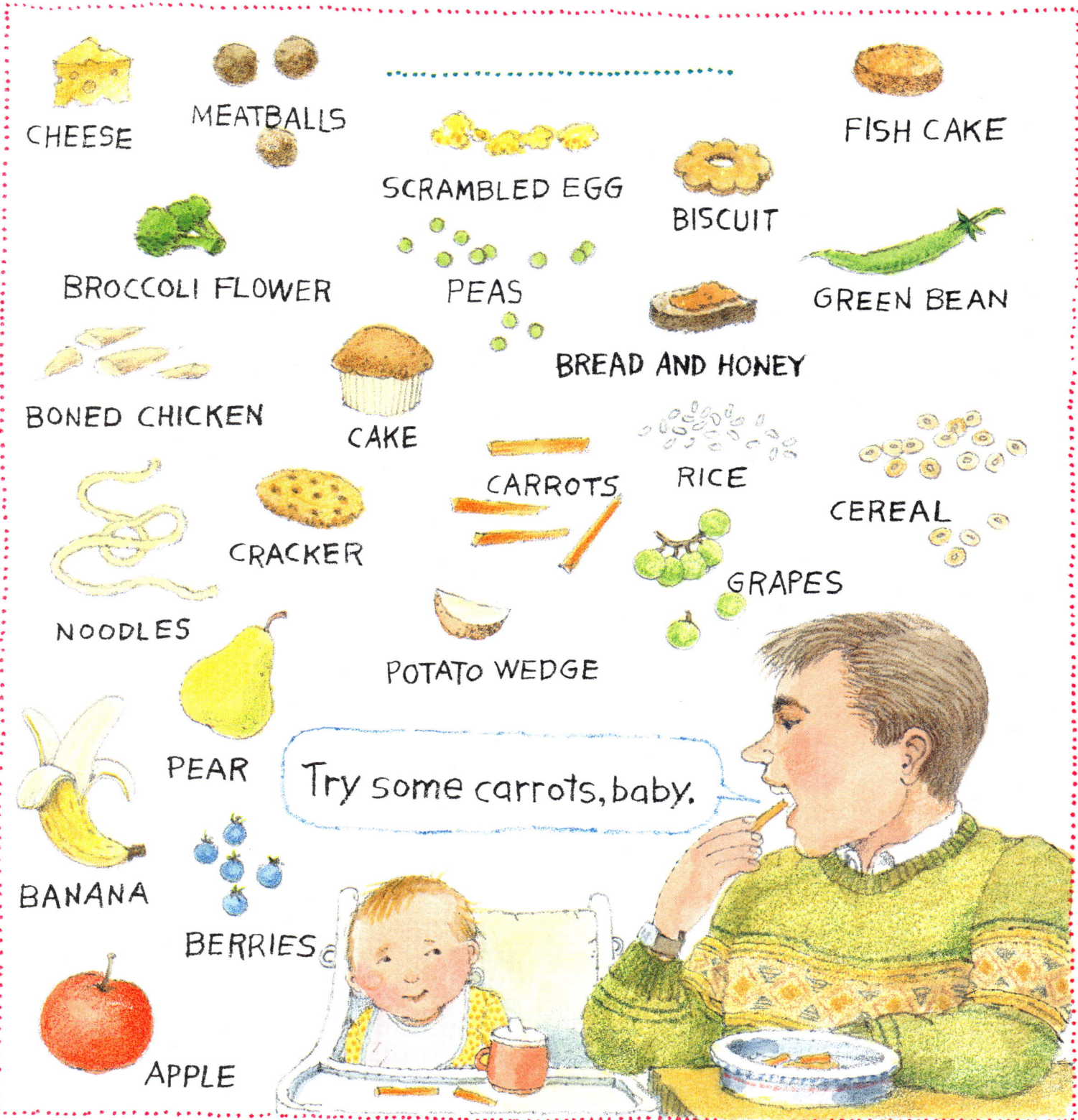

THINGS TO CHEW

You will find your baby gets to know something by putting it in her mouth. If you use a dummy, give your baby plenty of time without it. Make safe objects available. Objects must be unbreakable, too big to swallow, nontoxic, without sharp edges and with no parts that come off or can reach the back of her throat.

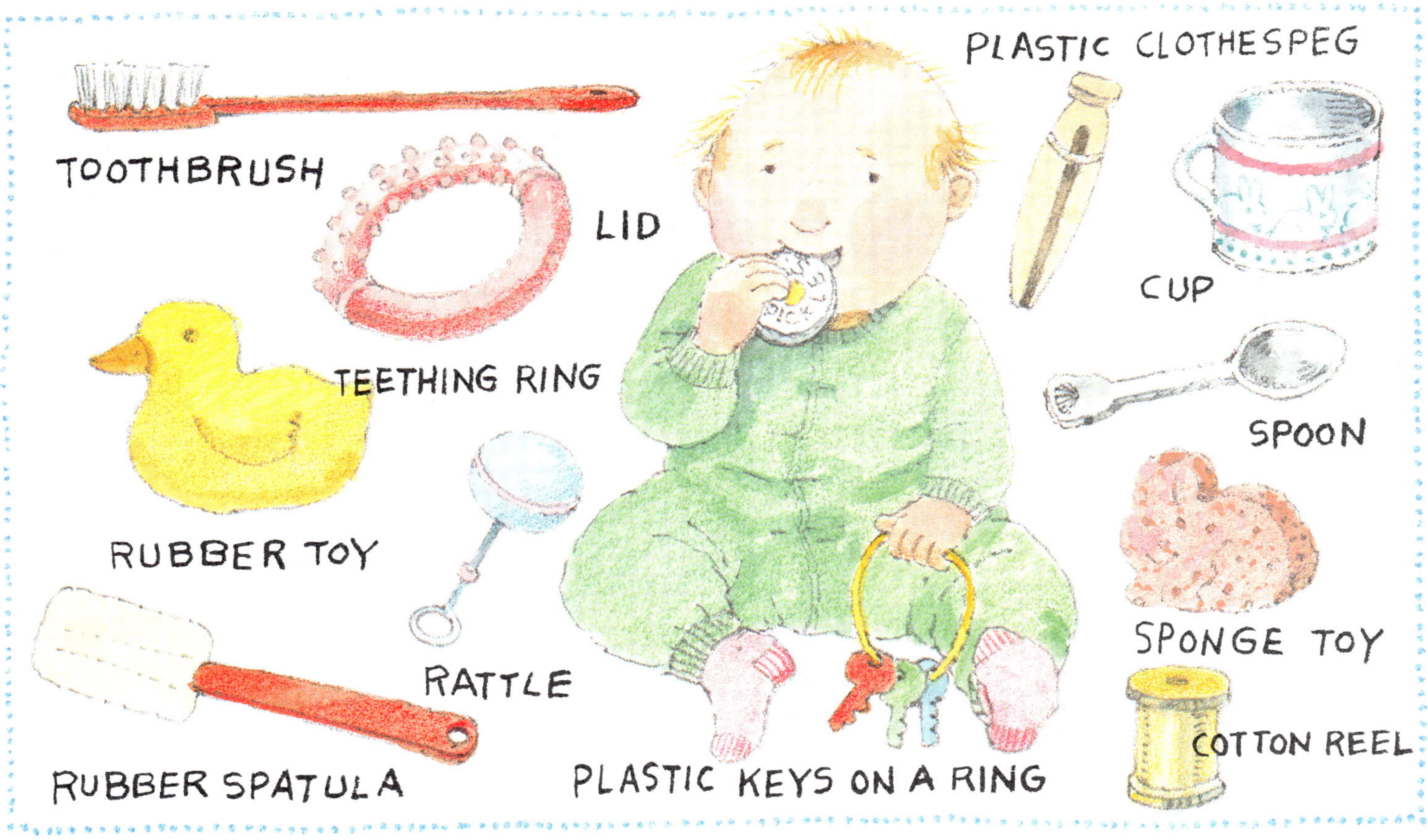

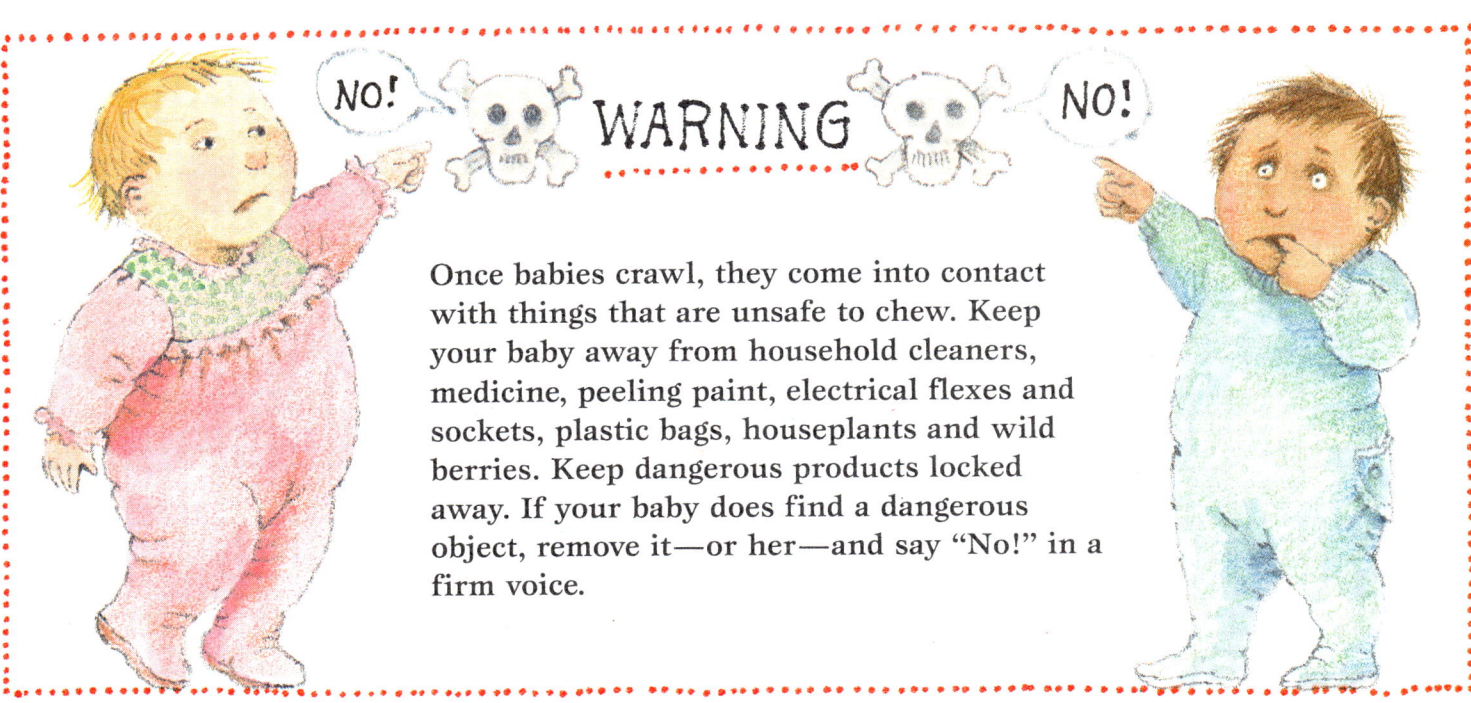

WARNING

Once babies crawl, they come into contact with things that are unsafe to chew. Keep your baby away from household cleaners, medicine, peeling paint, electrical flexes and sockets, plastic bags, houseplants and wild berries. Keep dangerous products locked away. If your baby does find a dangerous object, remove it—or her—and say "No!" in a firm voice.

TOUCH

Being in close physical contact with you comforts your baby and helps him feel safe. The more physically secure he feels, the more eager he will be to reach out and explore his surroundings.

As your baby learns to look forward to your cuddles and hugs, he will also begin returning your affection. Somehow, magically, all those sleepless nights seem a small price to pay for his love.

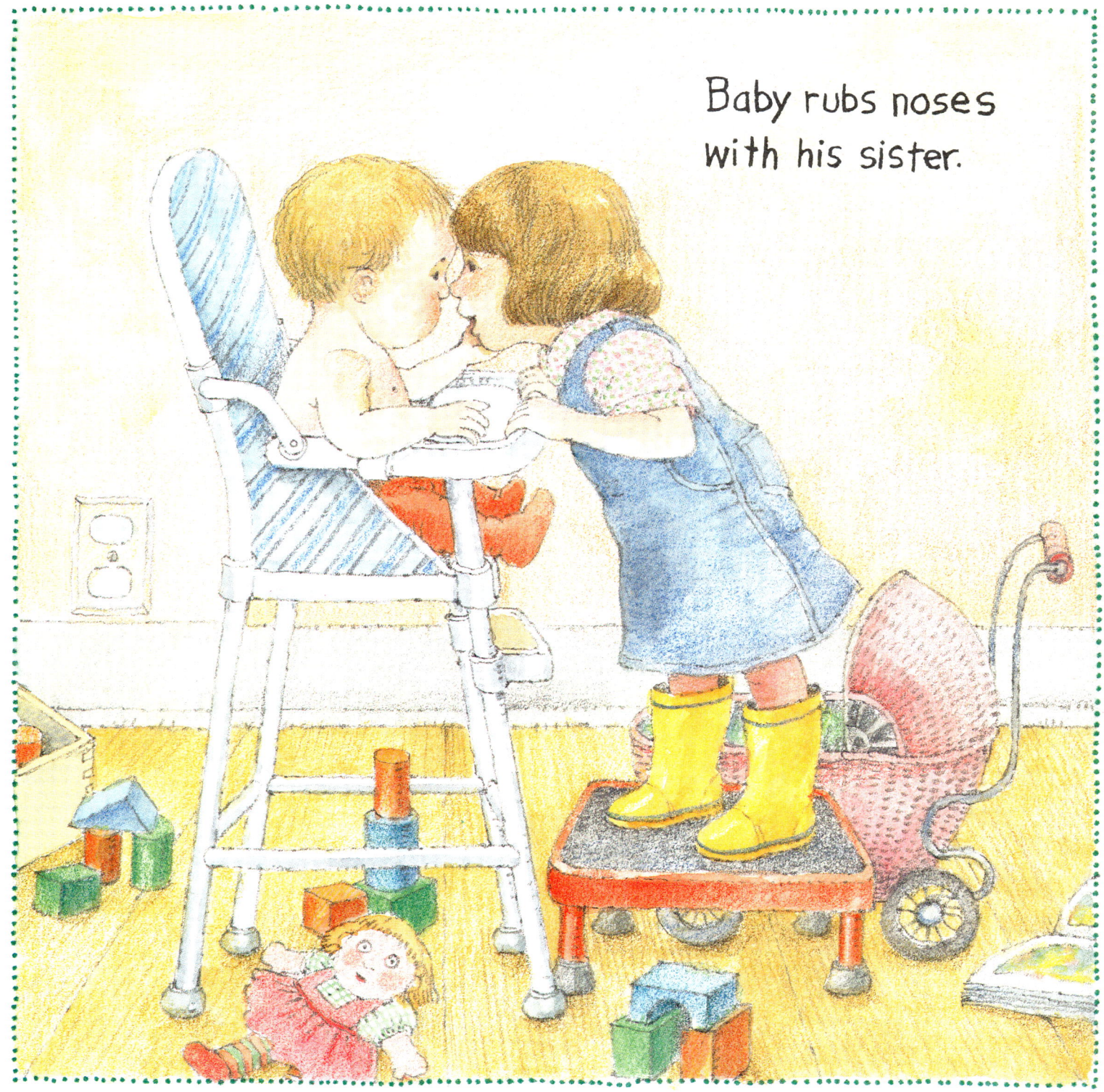

Baby rubs noses with his sister.

SELF-DISCOVERY

Babies feel warm or cold; they may hurt; they get hungry. They experience closeness with others. In time they become aware of their physical self: two hands, two feet, two ears, a tummy, perhaps hair.... They explore and try out their bodies.

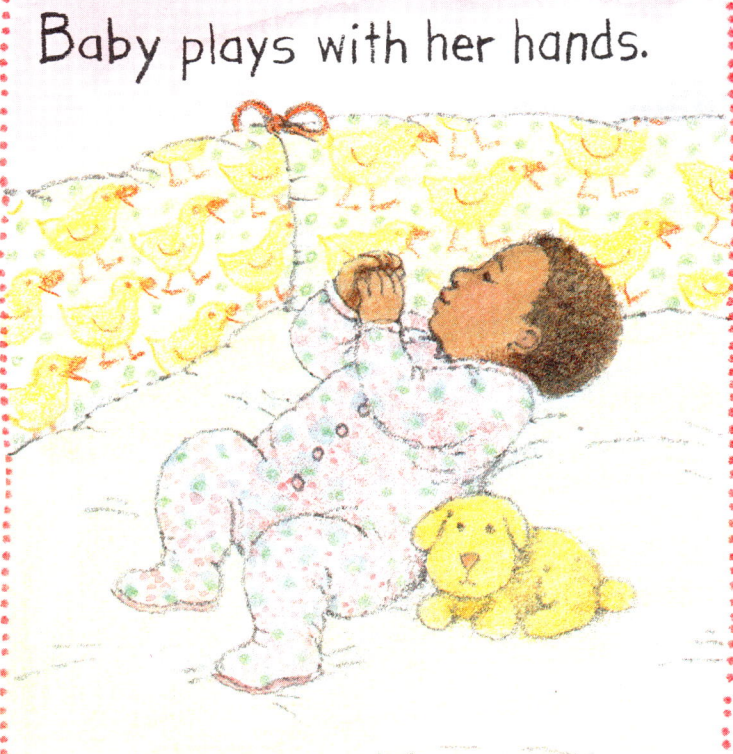

Baby plays with her hands.

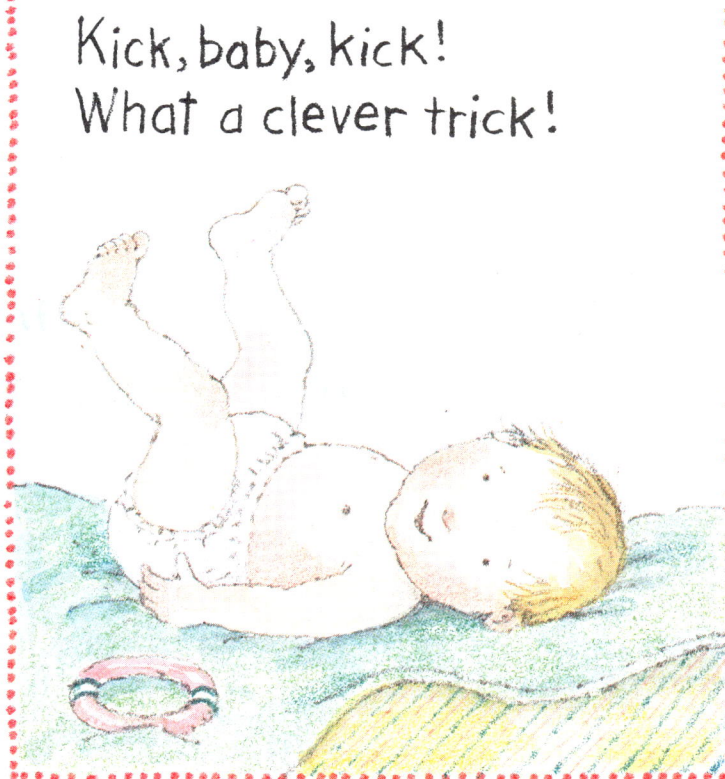

Kick, baby, kick!
What a clever trick!

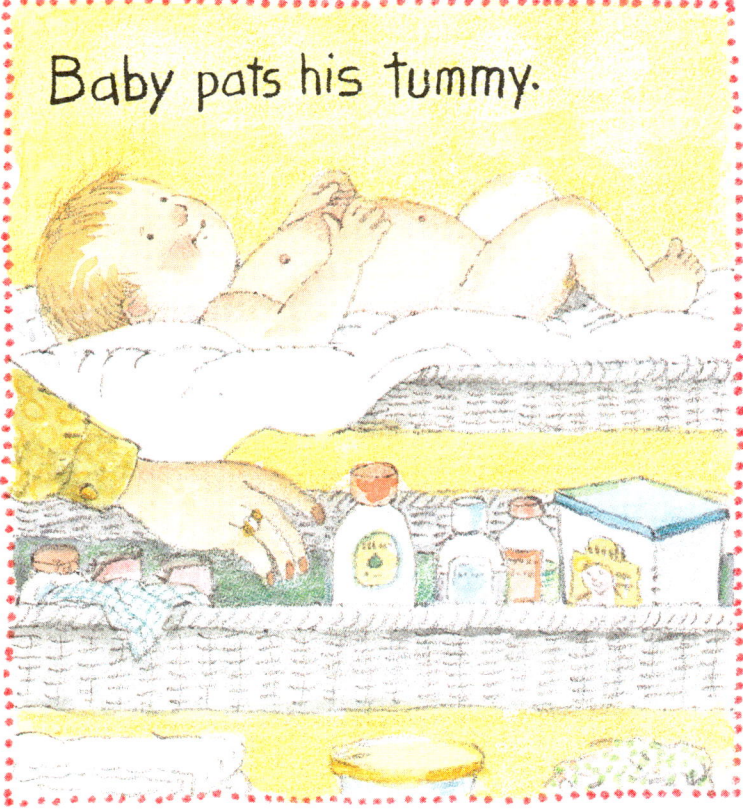

Baby pats his tummy.

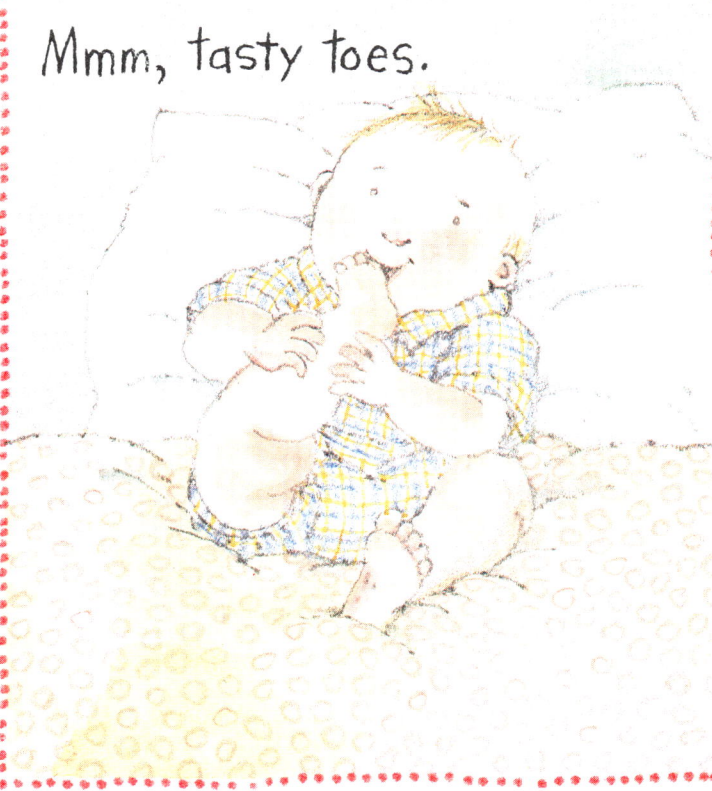

Mmm, tasty toes.

BATH TIME

Encourage your baby to play in her bath and enjoy the sensual feel of warm water, a firm sponge, tickly bubbles, a slippery ball and so on.

Very young babies need only their faces, hands, and bottoms washed every day. Introduce your baby gradually to bathing in a small tub and don't worry if she resists once in a while.

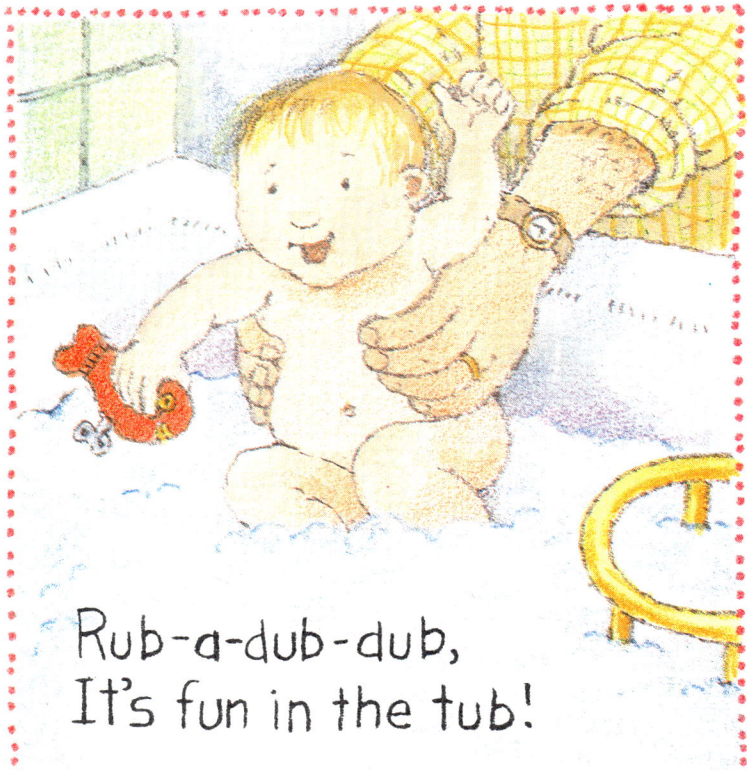

Rub-a-dub-dub,
It's fun in the tub!

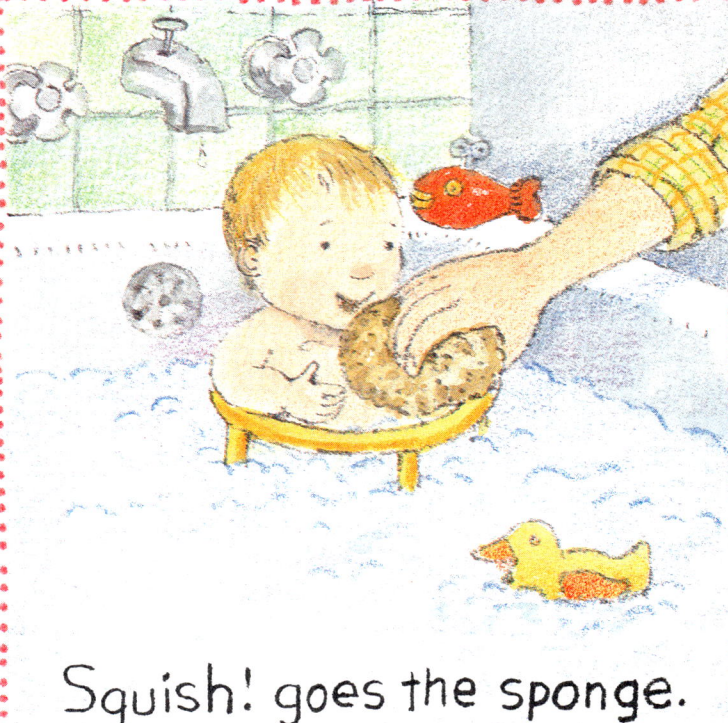

Squish! goes the sponge.

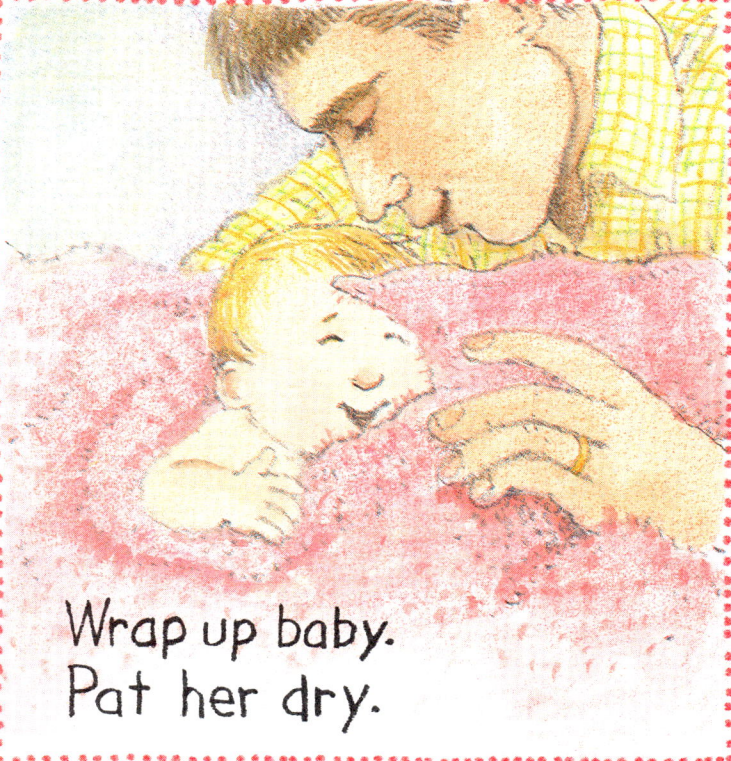

Wrap up baby.
Pat her dry.

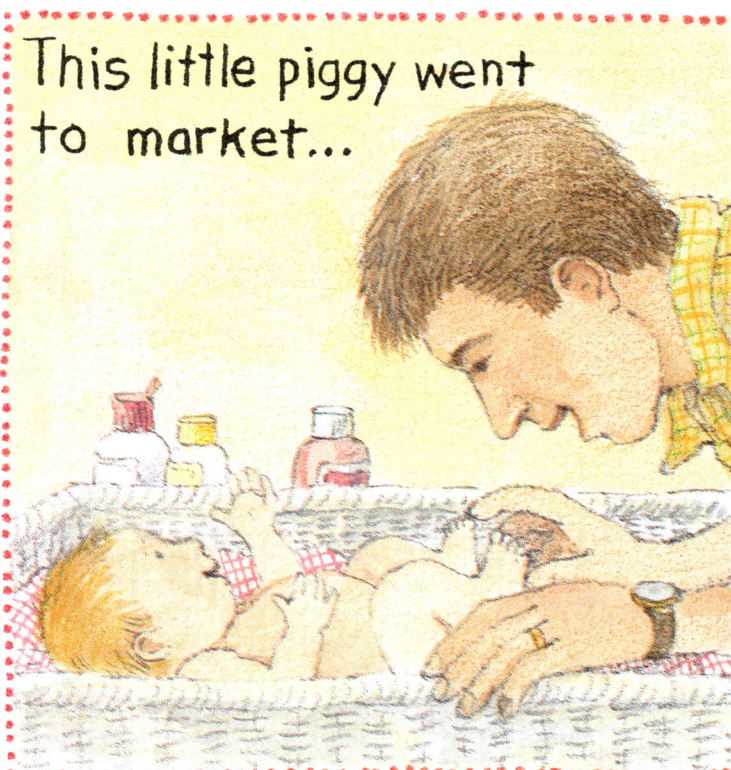

This little piggy went to market...

STROKING AND TOUCHING

Babies can enjoy and benefit from being touched and stroked. It relaxes their muscles, exercises joints, promotes body awareness, and helps develop a close relationship between the baby and whoever cares for him.

Vary your touch and try to keep your movements slow and rhythmic by relaxing and taking your time.

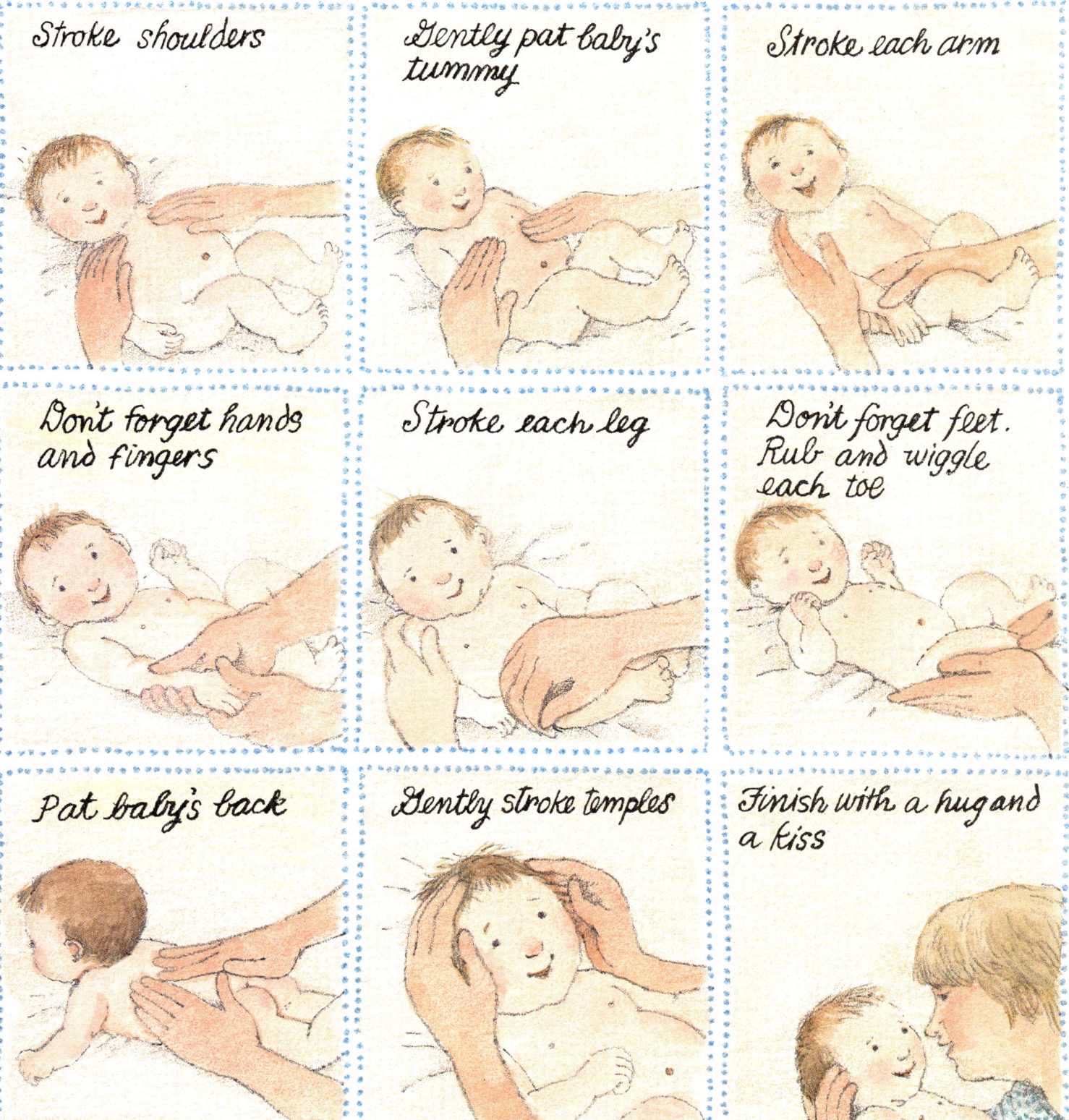

TOUCHING OTHERS

Your baby will learn how to touch others by the way you handle him. Let him know if he hurts you unintentionally. Showing your baby how to be considerate of living things helps him learn to be loving and kind.

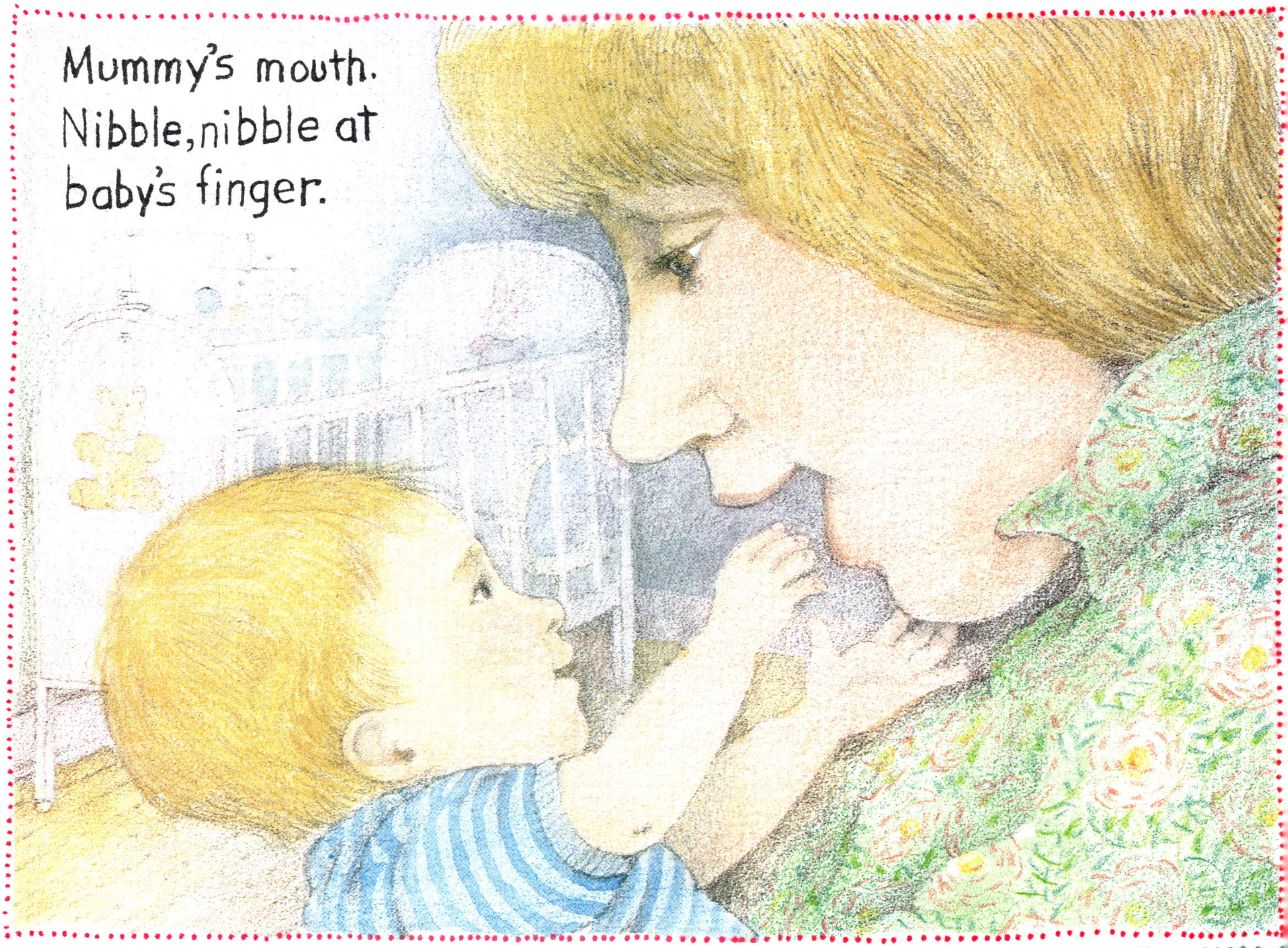

Mummy's mouth. Nibble, nibble at baby's finger.

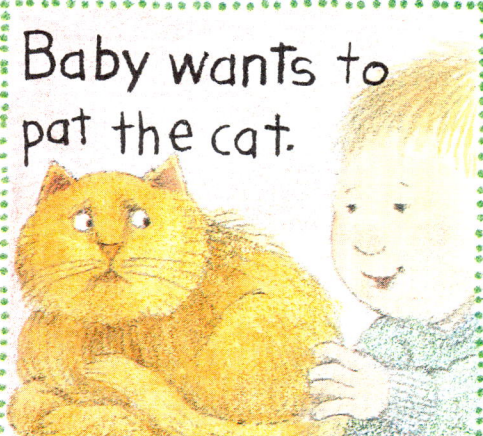

Baby wants to pat the cat.

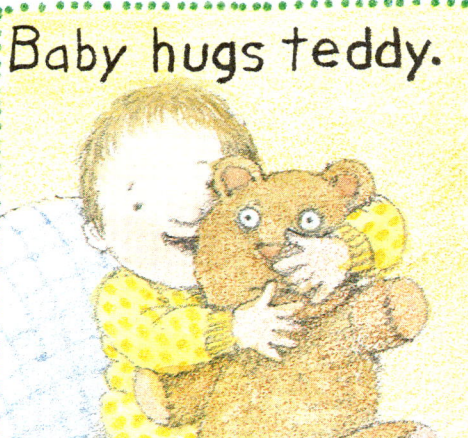

Baby hugs teddy.

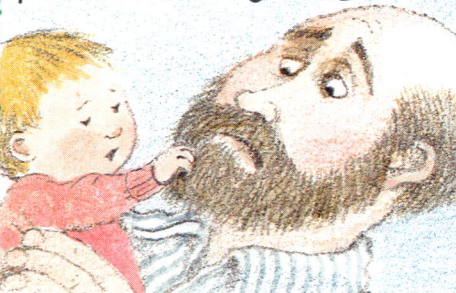

No, no, baby. Don't pull uncle's beard.

THINGS TO TOUCH

Let your baby discover different textures by touching and comparing opposite things that are smooth or rough, hard or soft, wet or dry. Make him aware of a thing's shape, temperature, and weight.

Babies love to handle paper. Let your baby tear, rustle, crumple, and study paper to his heart's content. (But be sure he doesn't swallow any!)

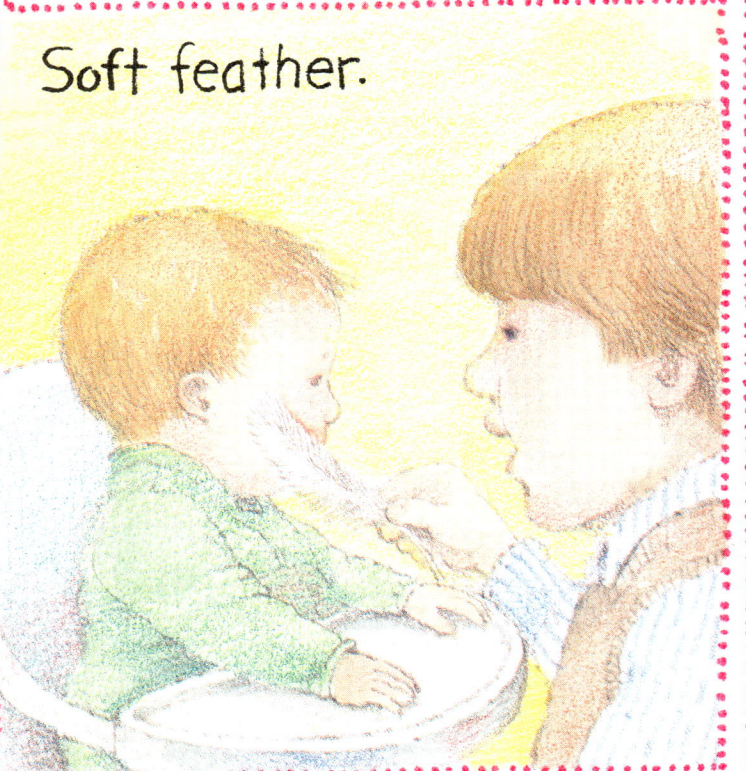

Soft feather.

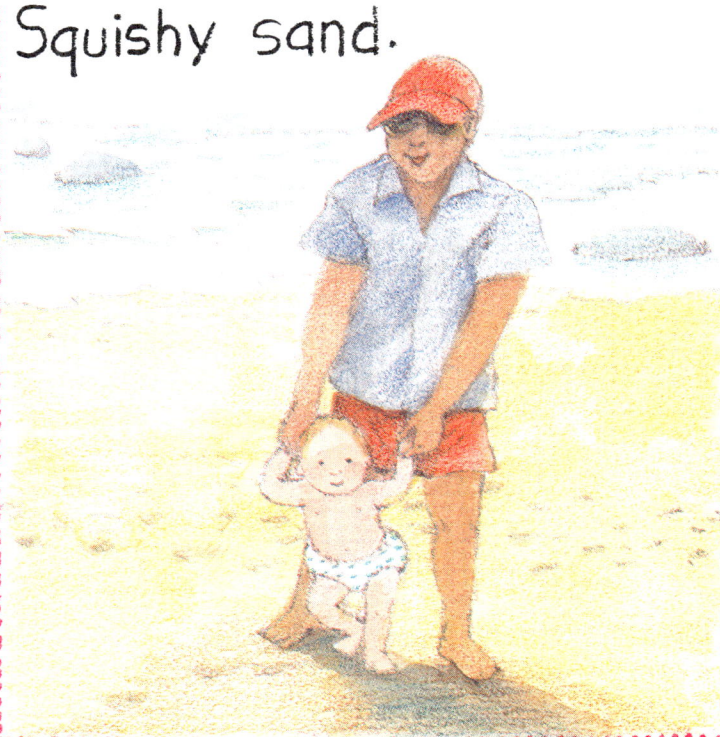

Squishy sand.

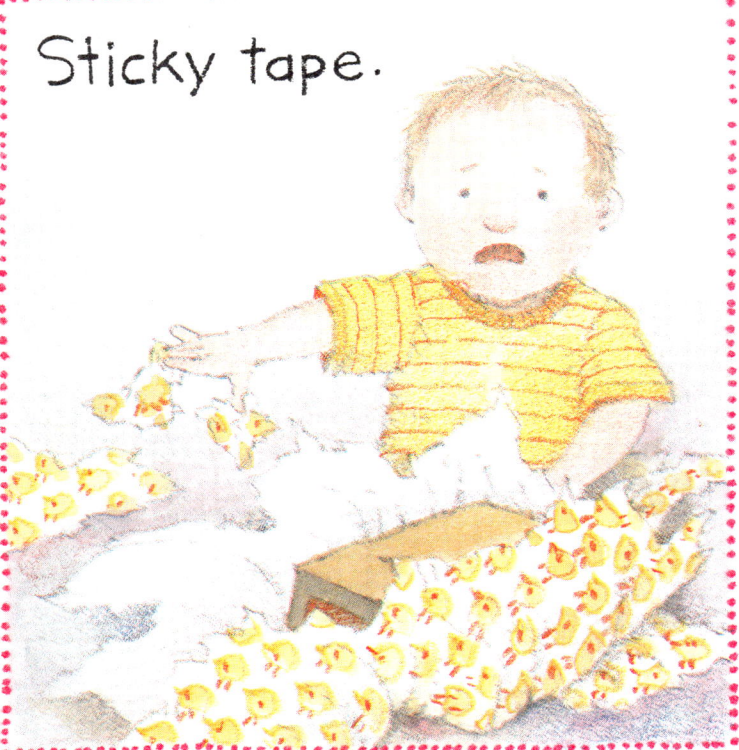

Sticky tape.

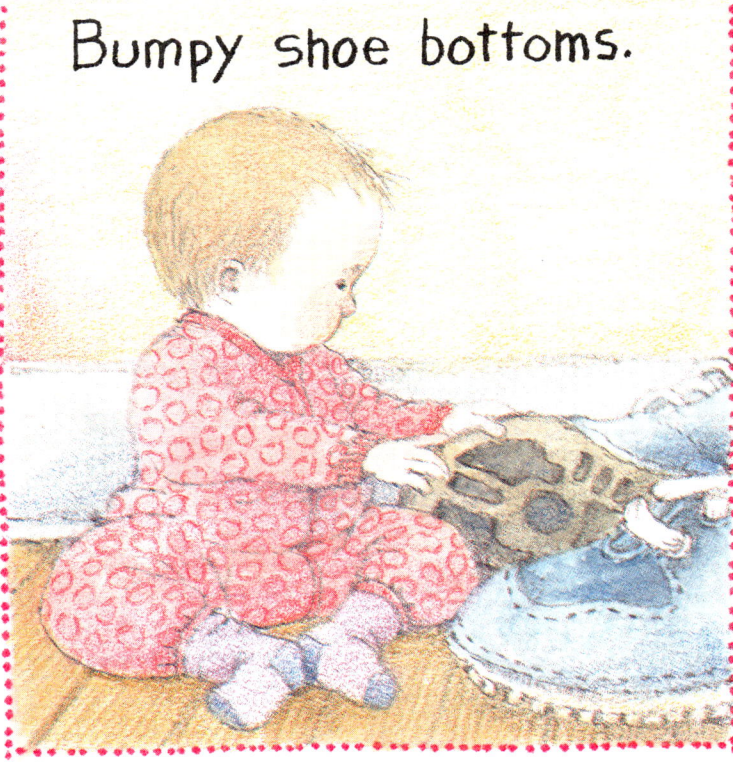

Bumpy shoe bottoms.

MOVEMENT

Carrying your baby in a sling lets her enjoy your body warmth and heartbeat and the motion of your footsteps—while you have both hands free!

Your baby will take her first steps when she is ready. She will want to practise often. You can help by providing safe spaces, sturdy things to hold on to, and patience to let her explore.

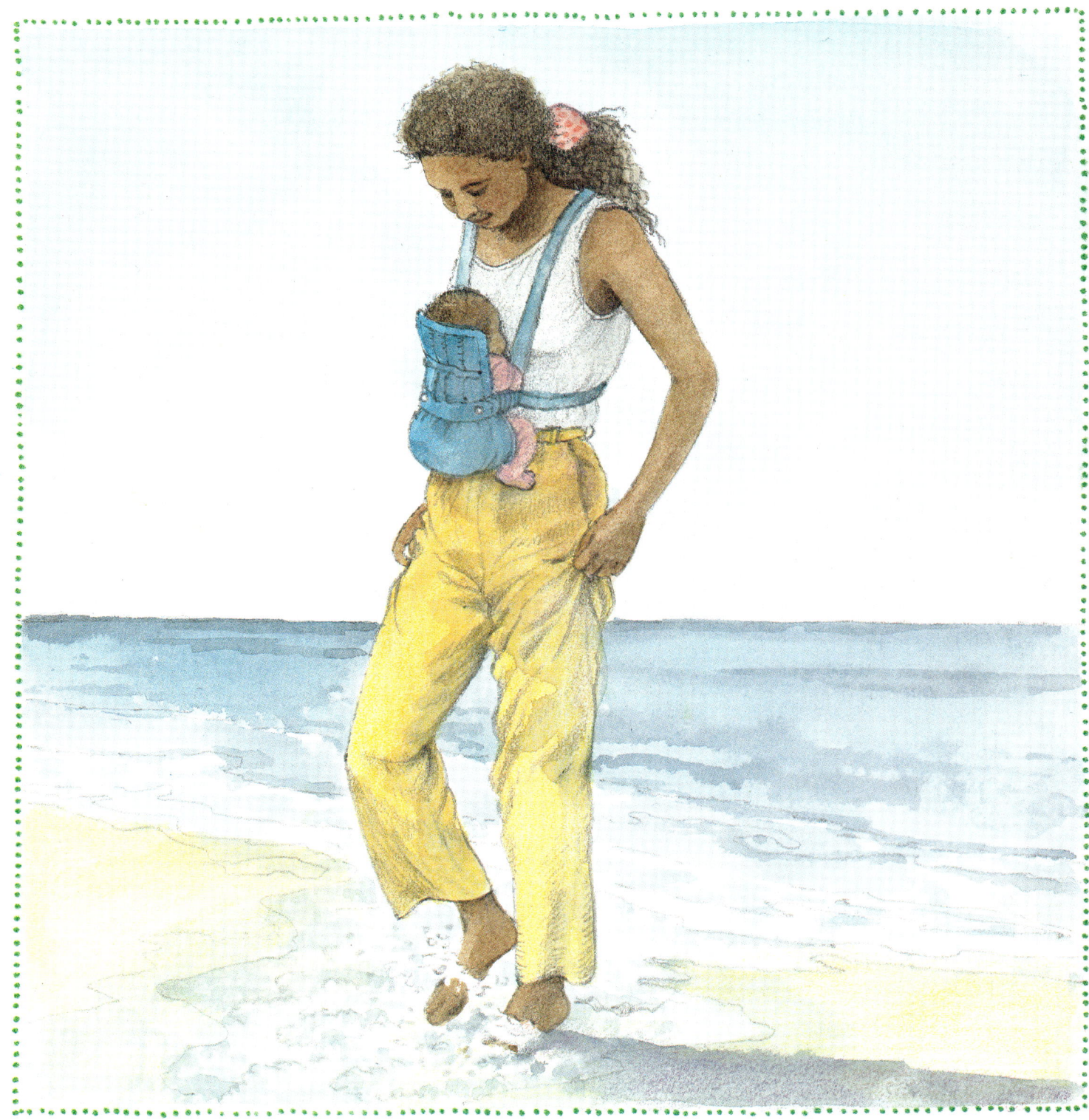

WAYS TO TRAVEL

There are many ways to transport your baby from place to place. Choose the one that is most convenient and pleasant for the situation.

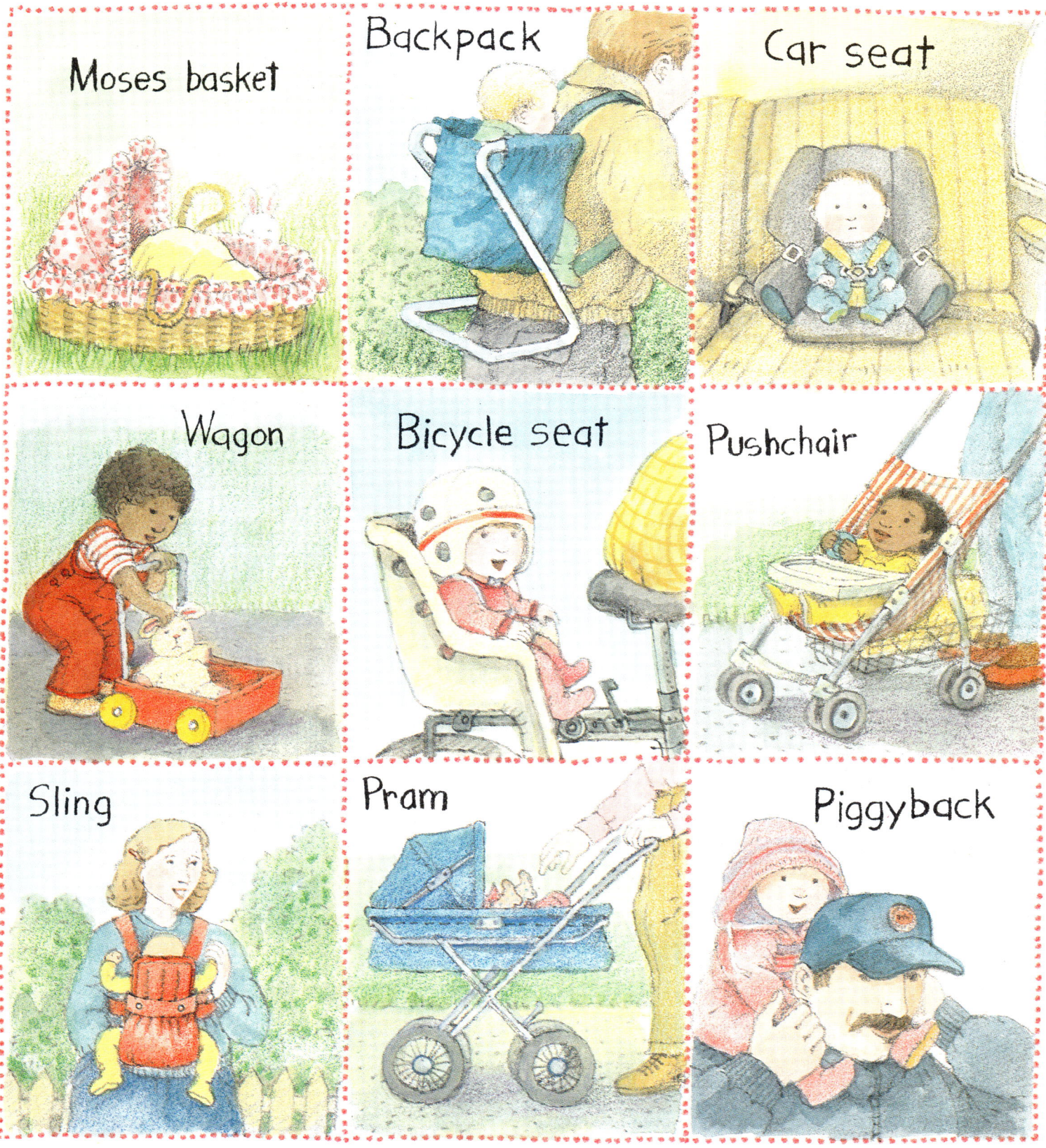

MOVING WITH HELP

Physical movement can soothe or stimulate your baby, so be aware of what sorts of activities you introduce. Balance boisterous play with gentle cuddling. After a long time in the pushchair, an older baby may welcome the chance to crawl around.

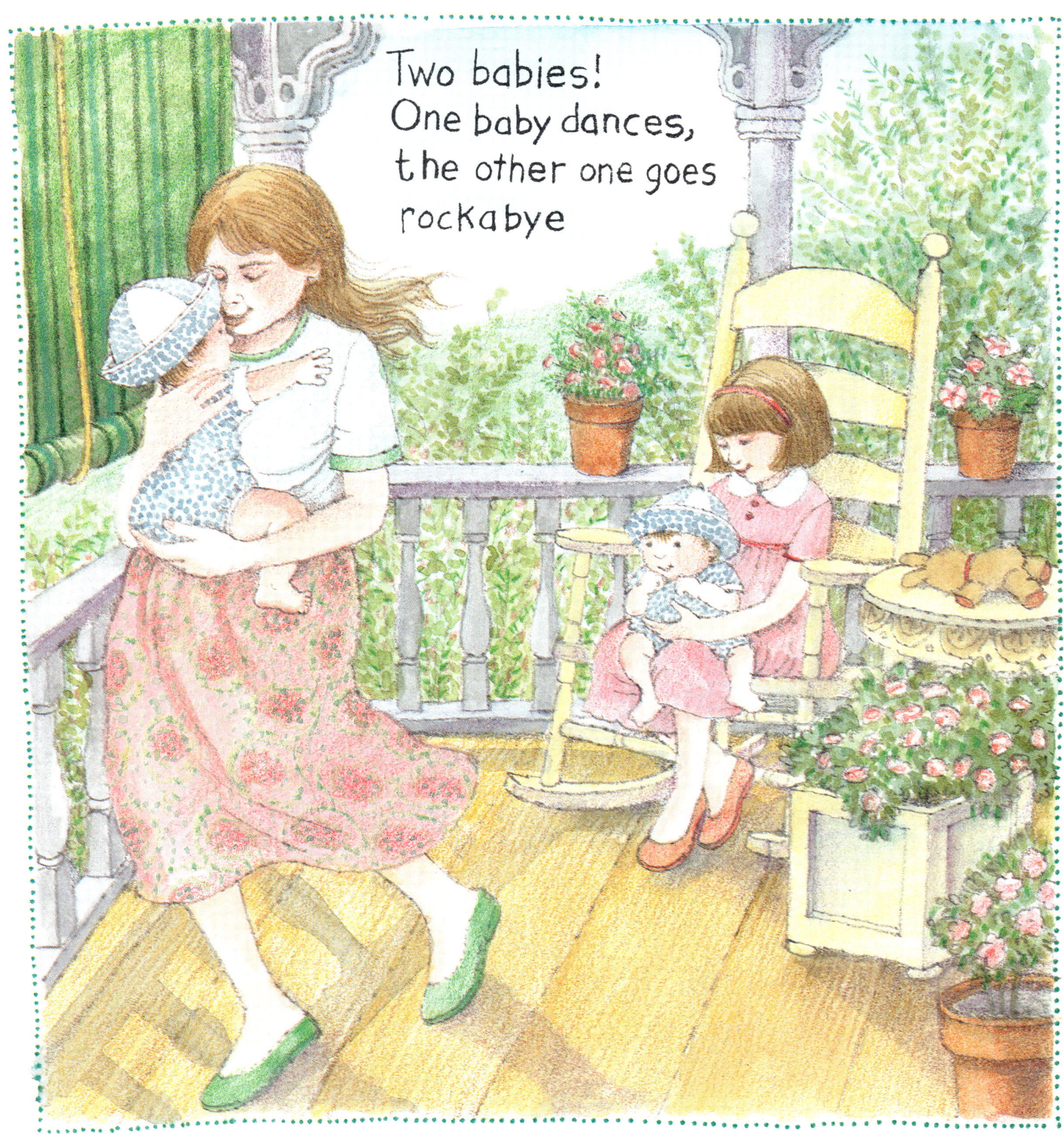

Two babies! One baby dances, the other one goes rockabye

MOVING WITH RHYME

Treat your baby to action rhymes. Babies enjoy both the feel of rhythmic motions and the sound of rhyming words. It is a winning combination for children, and one that helps both physical and language development. Repeat the rhymes your baby especially likes; there is added pleasure in going through familiar motions again and again.

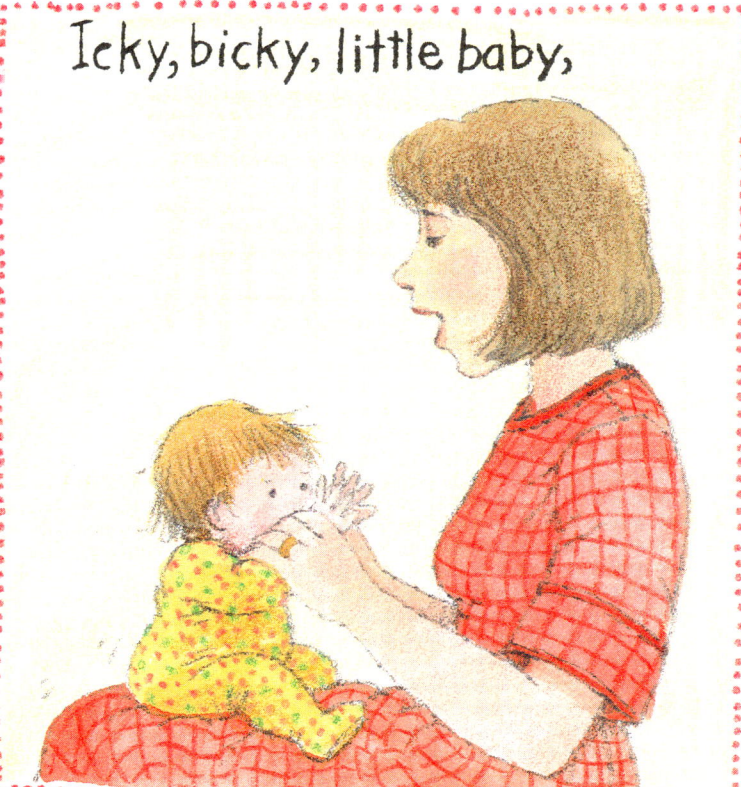

Icky, bicky, little baby,

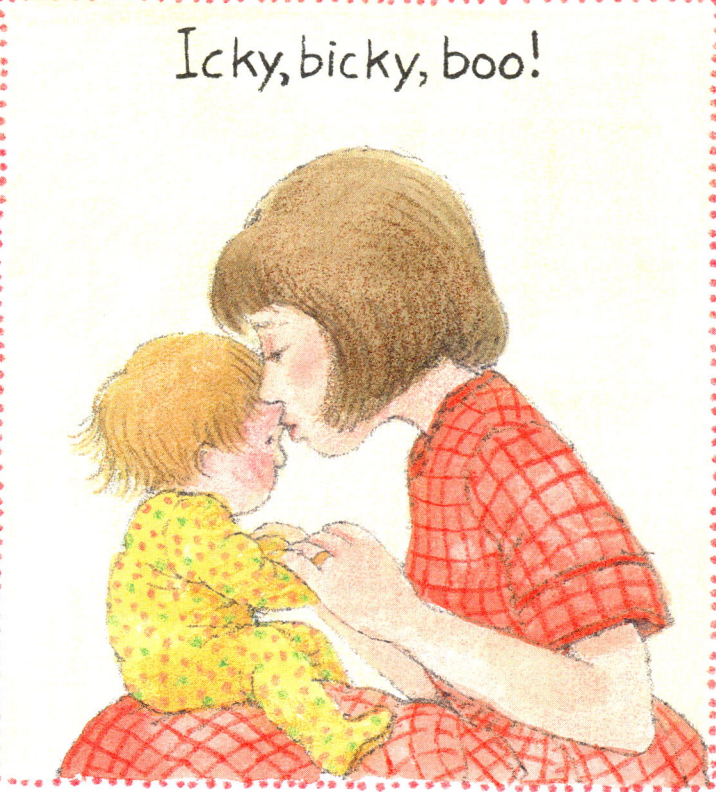

Icky, bicky, boo!

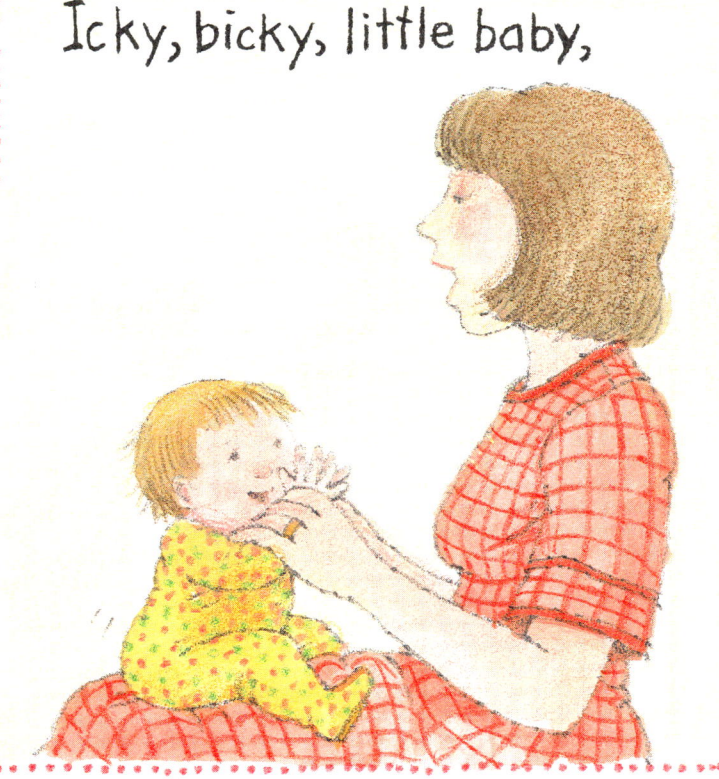

Icky, bicky, little baby,

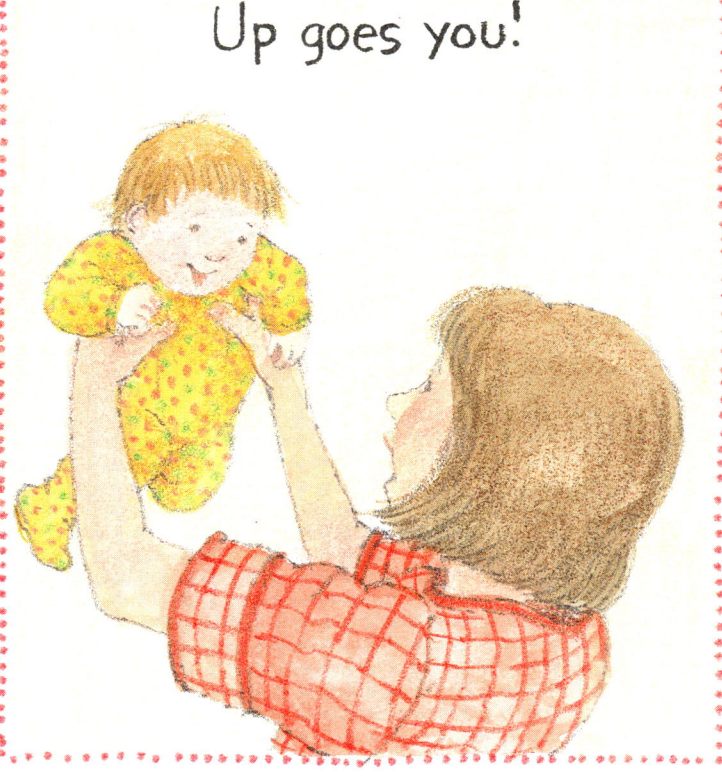

Up goes you!

ACTIONS

Allow your baby more and more opportunities to act independently. By watching her, you can judge when to offer help and when to let her try doing things herself. Encourage her to keep trying, if only for another minute. Praise good effort as well as success.

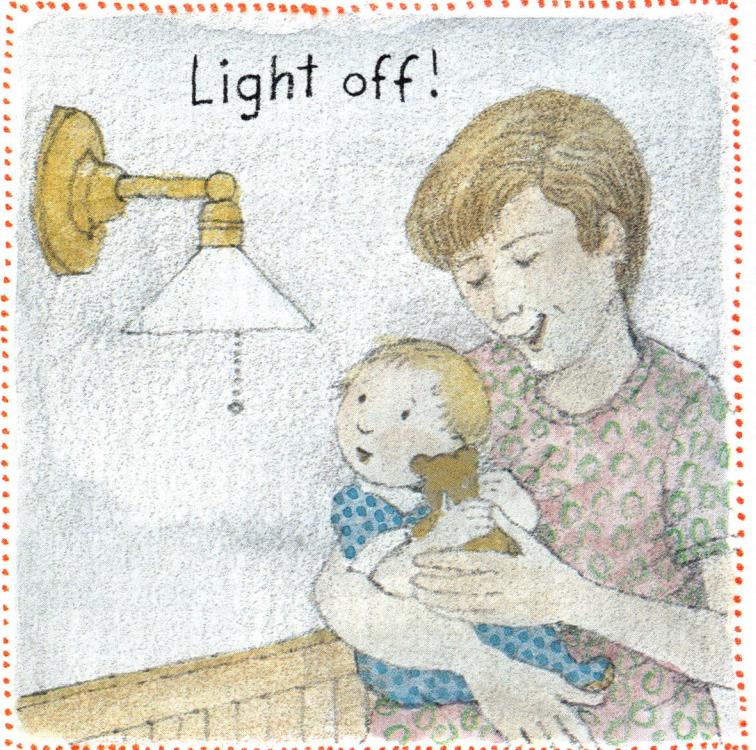

Light off!

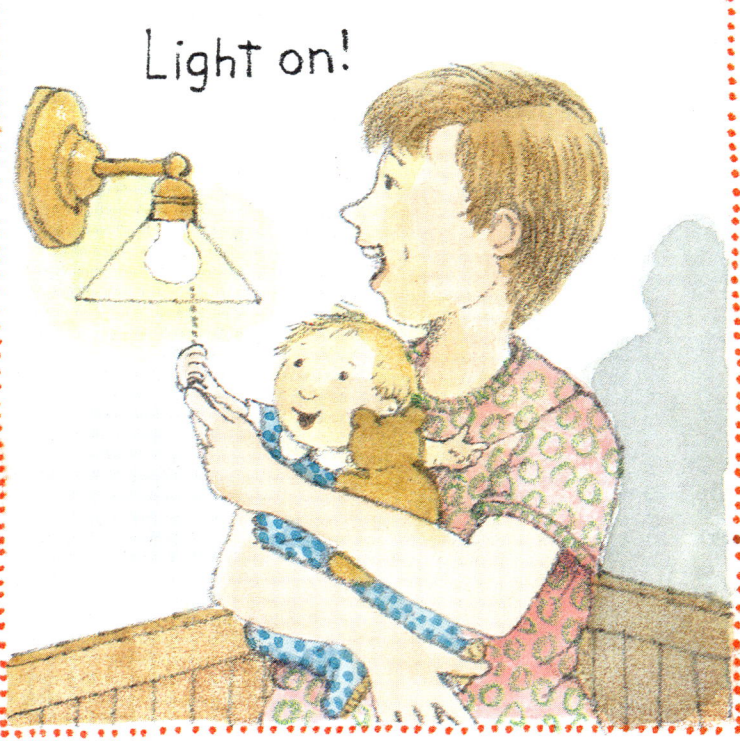

Light on!

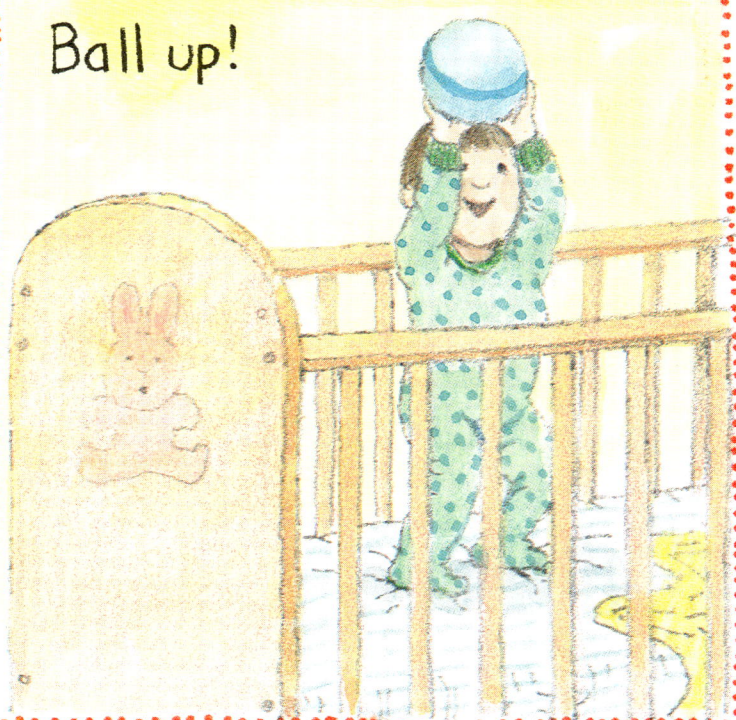

Ball up!

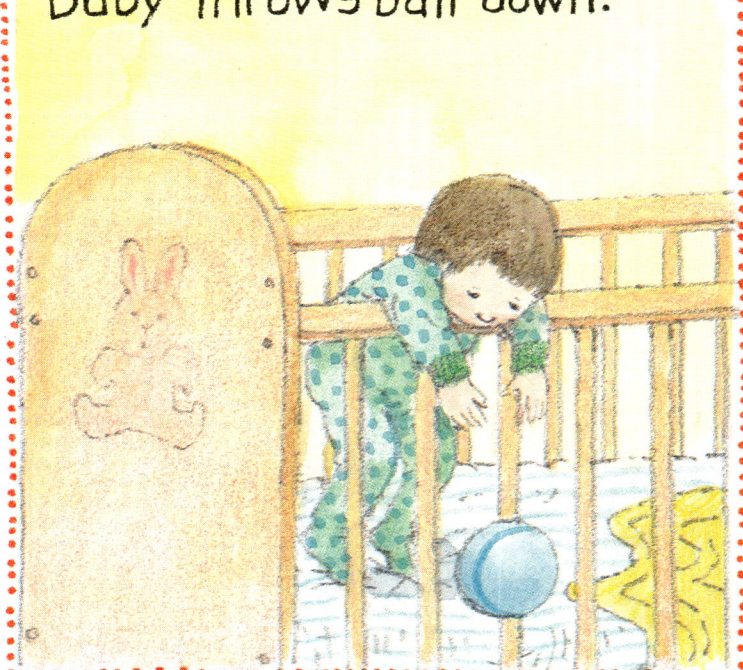

Baby throws ball down!

ACTIONS

Don't be discouraged when your baby starts to empty shelves and drawers. First she enjoys just taking things out; later she will learn to replace them.

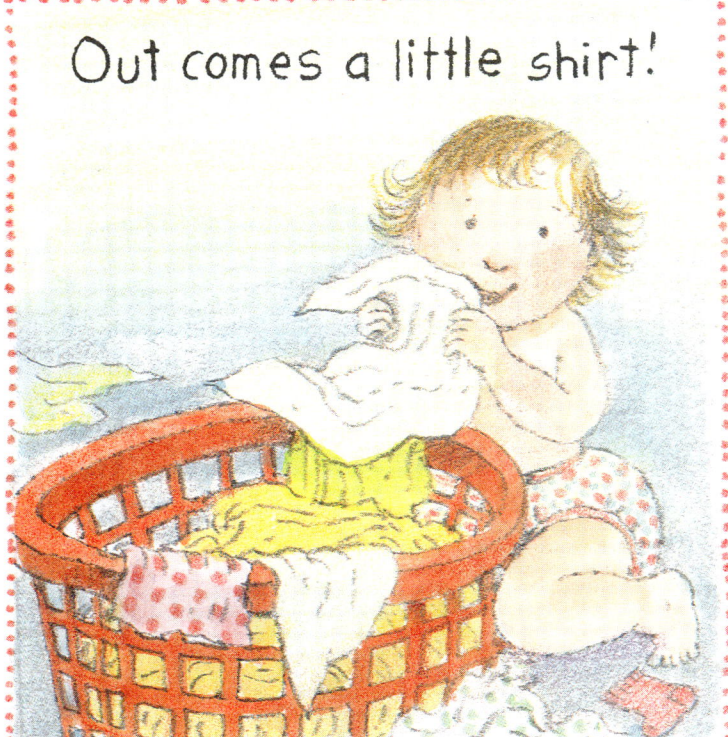

Out comes a little shirt!

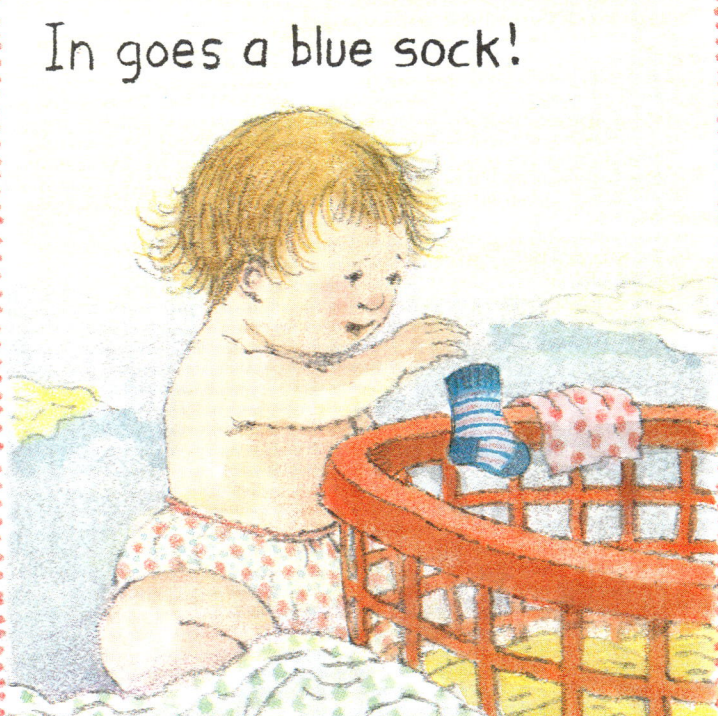

In goes a blue sock!

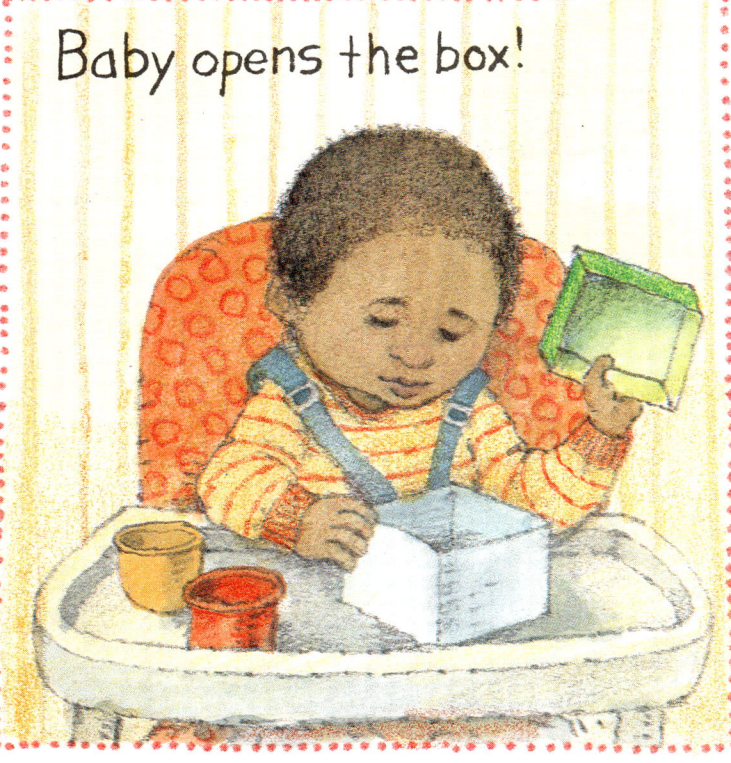

Baby opens the box!

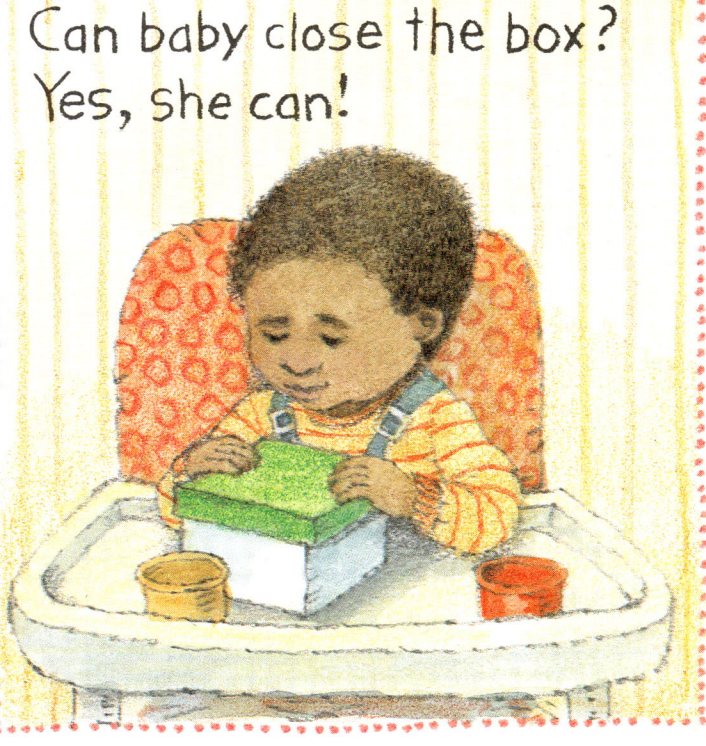

Can baby close the box? Yes, she can!

IMITATION

Babies learn a great deal from watching and trying to copy what the people around them do. Show your baby how to comb his hair or put a toy back on the shelf. To him, practising such simple tasks is more play than hard work, and it will teach him responsible behaviour. Be careful what you do in front of his curious eyes, though; he may also imitate behaviour you didn't intend him to learn!

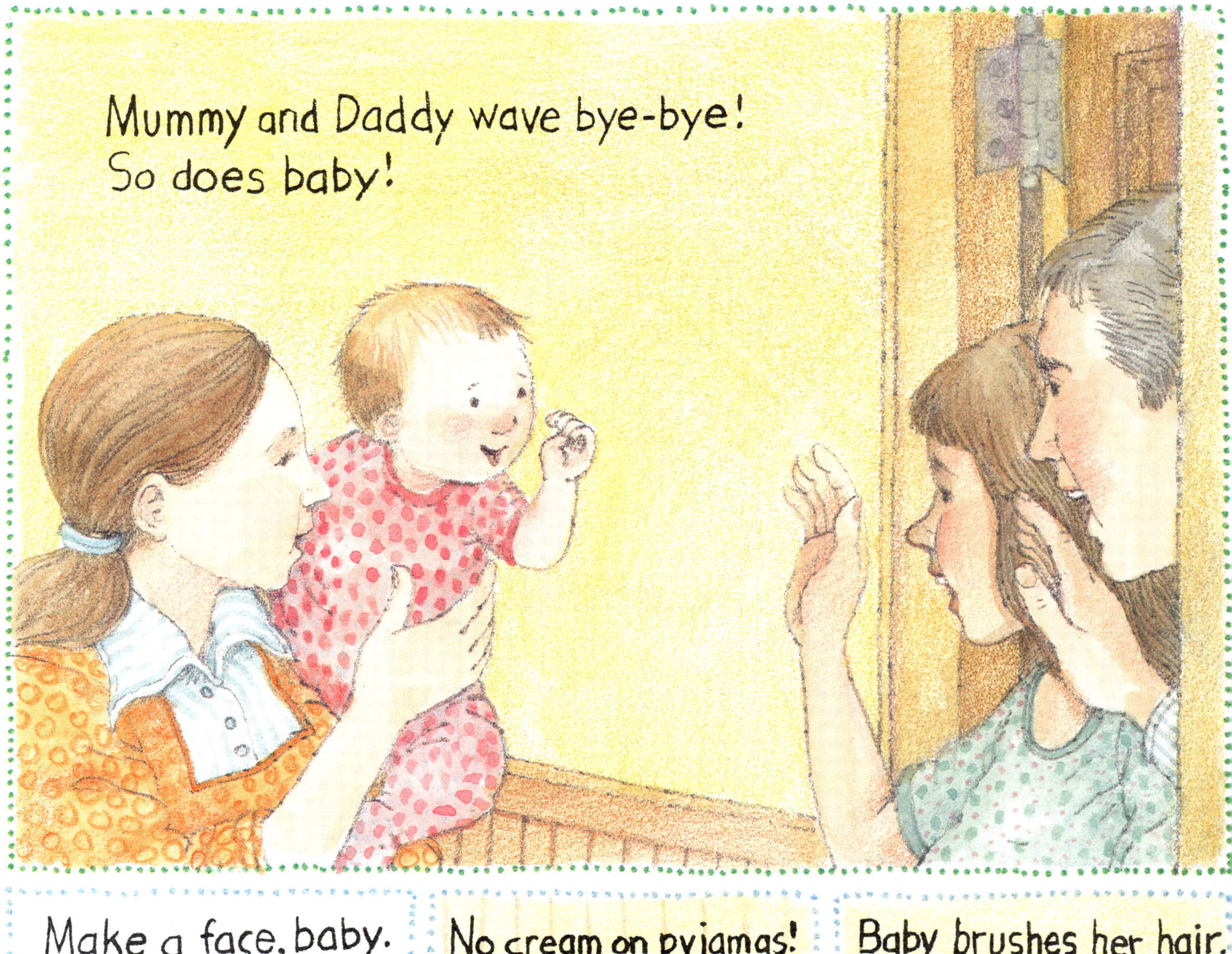

Mummy and Daddy wave bye-bye! So does baby!

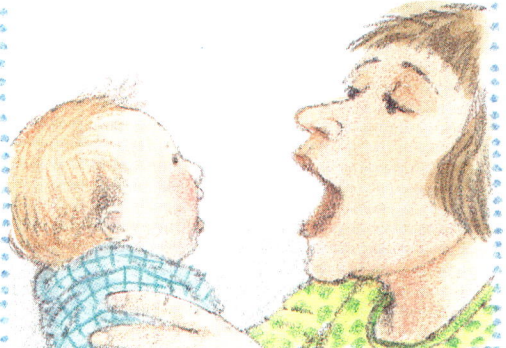
Make a face, baby.

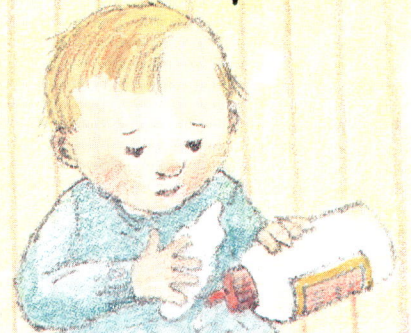
No cream on pyjamas!

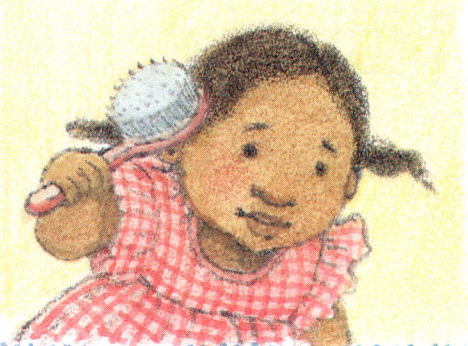
Baby brushes her hair.

PHYSICAL MILESTONES

Every baby matures at his own rate. Enjoy each tiny step in your baby's development. Notice how his behaviour changes and celebrate his progress. There's no need to rush. Motor skills develop in a logical order that includes the following stages.

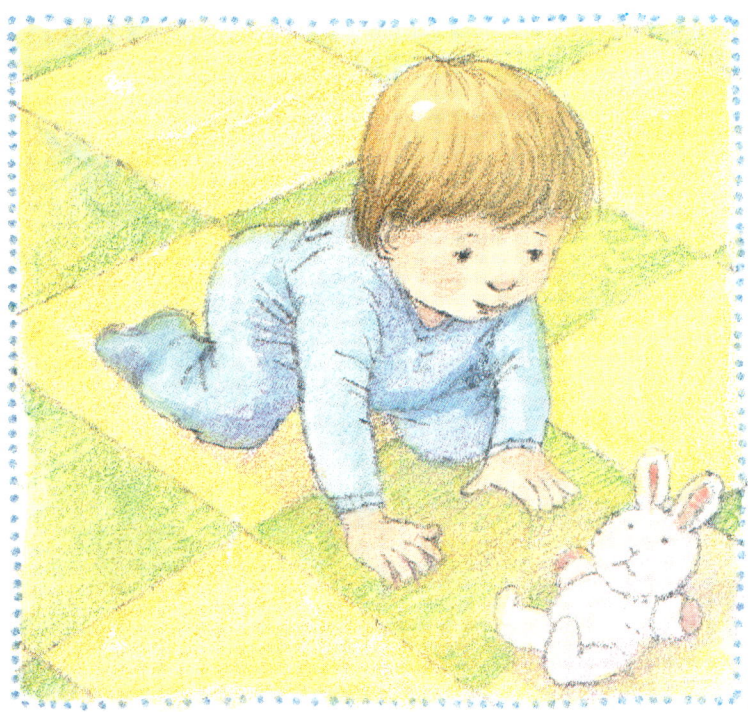 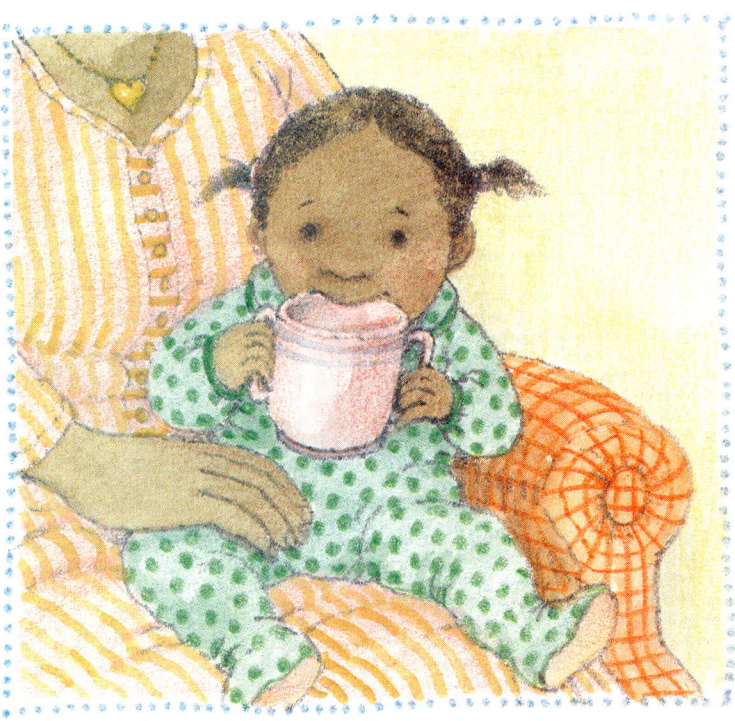

WHOLE BODY SKILLS

Holds up head
Sits supported
Rolls over
Rocks on hands and feet
Sits without support
Crawls or creeps
Pulls up to stand
Cruises holding on
Stands alone
First steps

HAND SKILLS

Grasps small object with palm and fingers
Reaches with two hands
Holds and shakes object with thumb and fingers
Reaches with one hand
Holds object with thumb and forefinger
Drops object on purpose
Transfers object hand to hand
Pokes with forefinger
Manipulates object

PLAYTHINGS

A baby's attention to most objects is short-lived. Select toys that interest your baby and help develop his skills in playing with them. Look around the house for safe things for your baby to handle. Household objects are often more fun for him than shop-bought toys. Mix and match objects. Rotate playthings by keeping some out of sight. Sell, save, give away, or discard toys as your baby outgrows them.

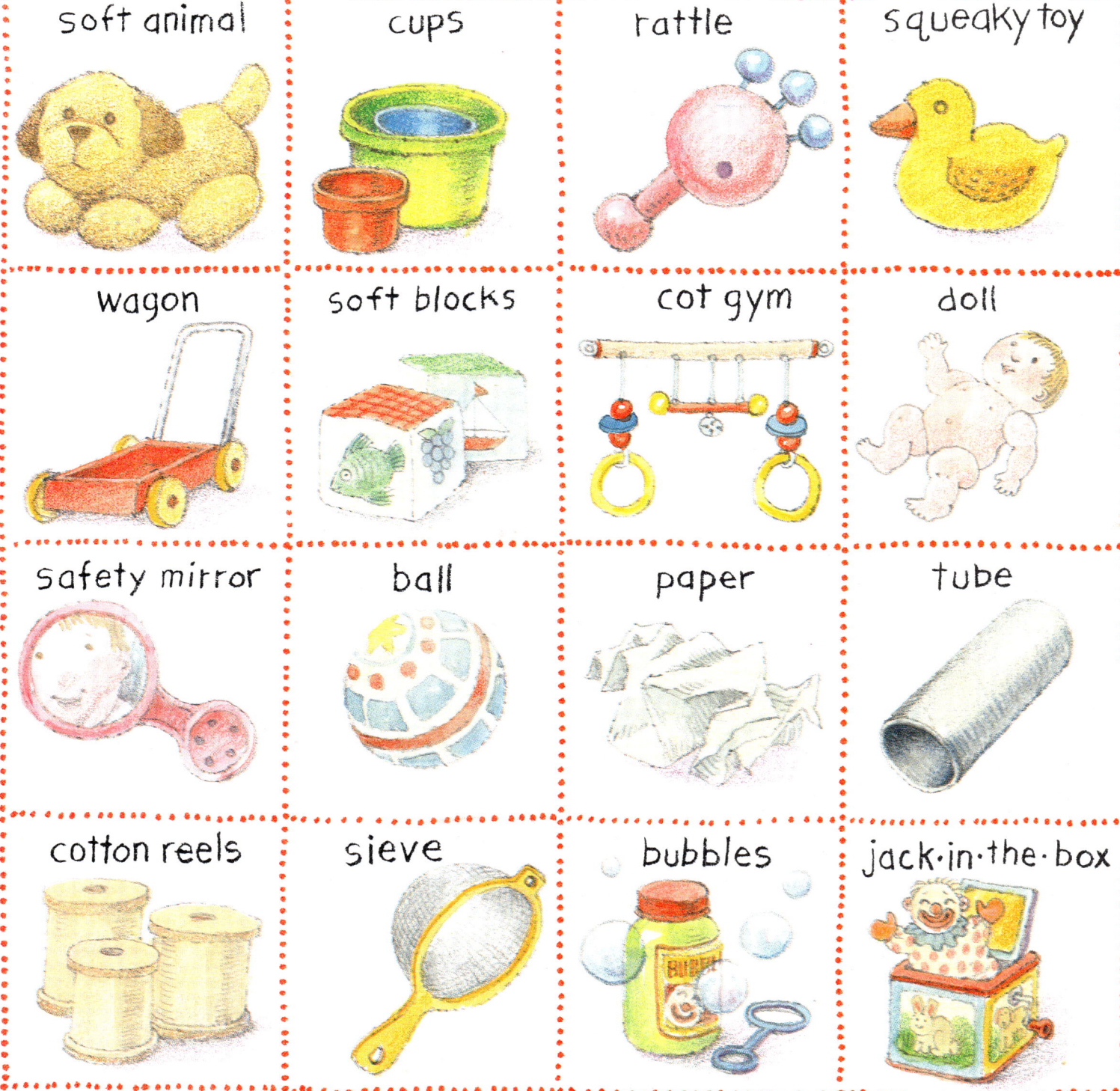

PLAYTHINGS

When you first give a new toy to your baby, show him how it works or what it can do.

From time to time, wash your baby's playthings in hot, soapy water.

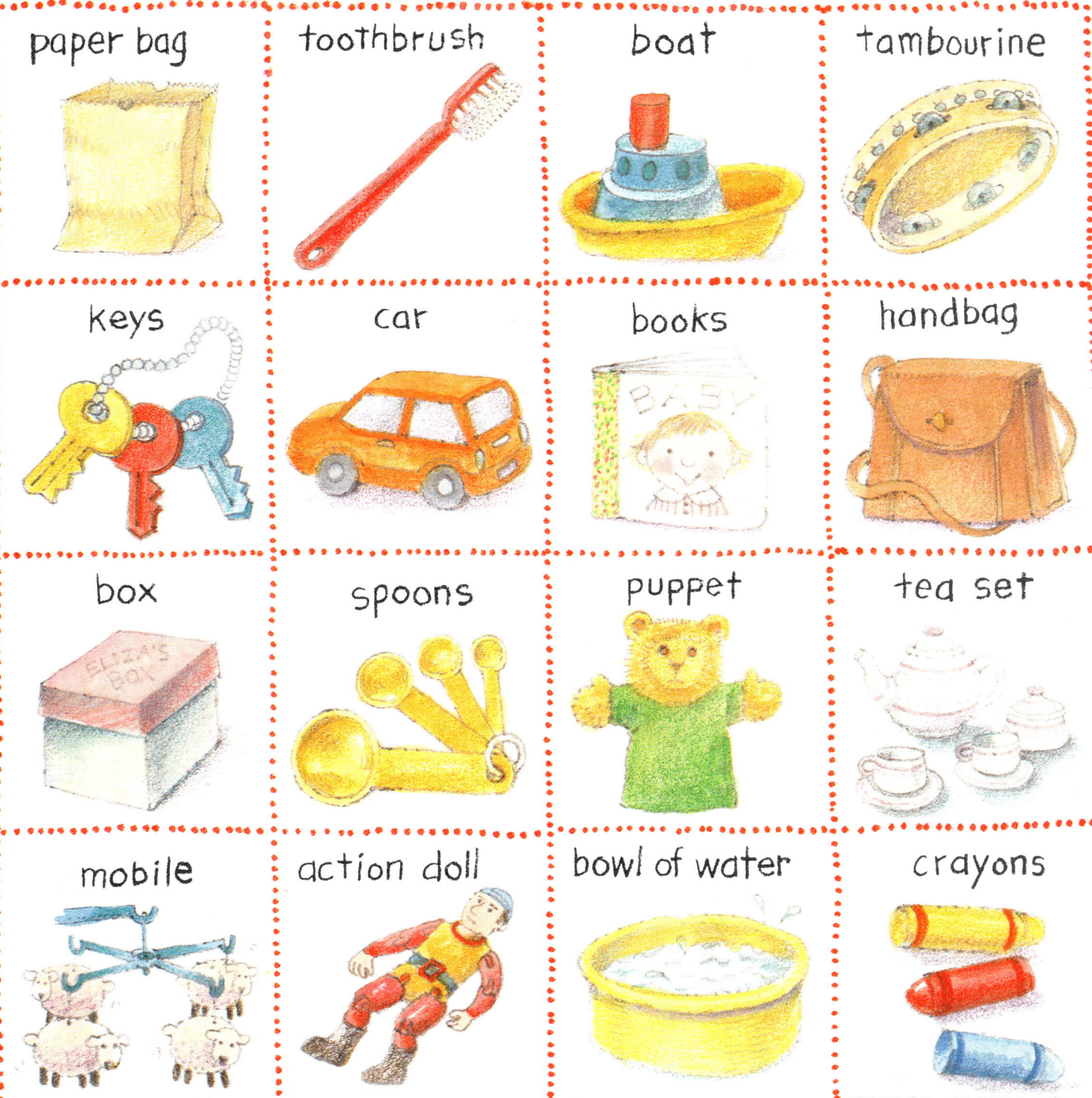

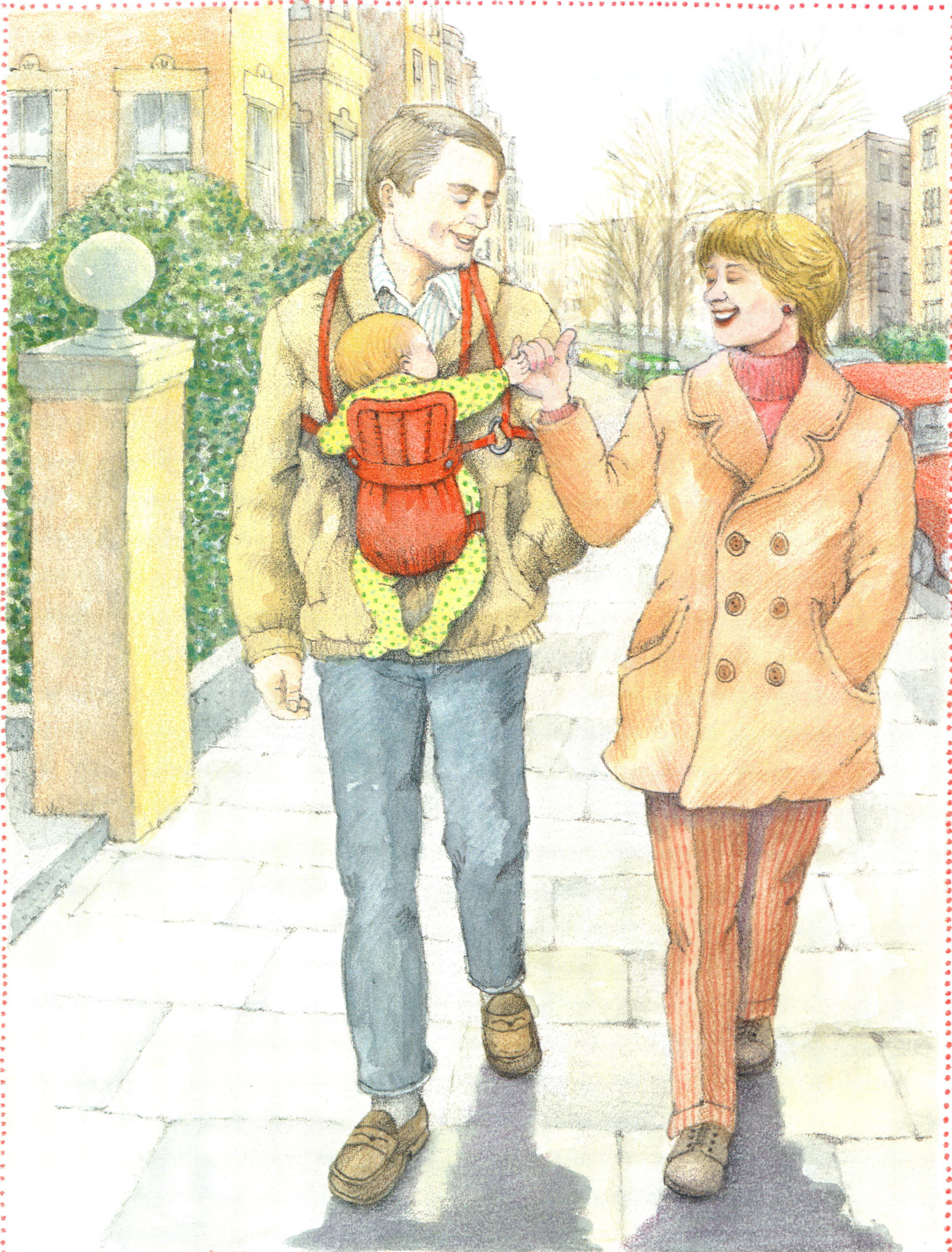

But one plaything is the favourite of all babies —
you!

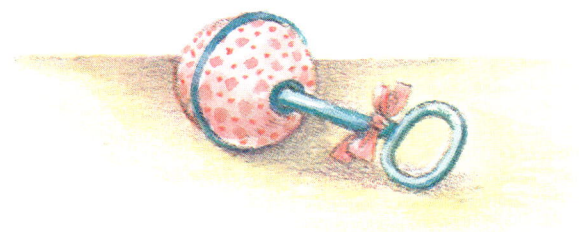